Plant Powered Health

Plant Powered Health

*The ultimate vegan starter guide to excellent health
and weight using the power of plants.*

LISA GOODWIN

Copyright © 2020 Lisa Goodwin

All Rights Reserved.

No part of this publication may be reproduced, distributed, or transmitted in any form or by any means, including photocopying, recording, or other electronic or mechanical methods, without the prior written permission of the publisher, except in the case of brief quotations embodied in critical reviews and certain other noncommercial uses permitted by copyright law.

Legal notice: Please note that much of this publication is based on personal experience. Although the author and editors made every reasonable attempt to achieve complete accuracy of the content in this product, they assume no responsibility for errors or omissions. This book is not intended to treat, cure, diagnose, or prevent any disease. It is not a substitute for medical advice from physicians. Consult your healthcare provider and follow all safety instructions before beginning any exercise program or nutrition plan.

The author: Lisa Goodwin

www.2sharemyjoy.com

lisagoodwin.business@gmail.com

Edited by: Terry Goodwin, B.A., English

To my husband-

Thank you for all of your insight, time, patience, and support while exploring the plant based lifestyle with me. Love you always.

Contents

INTRODUCTION: My Vegan Story — x

Part 1: Vegan Diet 101

CHAPTER 1: The Many Ways of Healthy — 2
CHAPTER 2: Reasons to Leverage the Power of Plants — 4
CHAPTER 3: Making Sense of Carbs, Protein, and Fat — 10
CHAPTER 4: Fiber, Pre-, and Probiotics — 20
CHAPTER 5: Mastering Micronutrients — 27
CHAPTER 6: Balancing your Meals — 46
CHAPTER 7: The 6 Hidden Troublemakers — 53
CHAPTER 8: Calories, Calories, Calories — 69
CHAPTER 9: Filled & Fueled Fat Loss — 73
CHAPTER 10: Plant Powered Muscle Gain — 78

Part 2: Transitioning In 3 Phases

PHASE 1: Add and Reduce — 82
Determining the Foods to Add and Reduce — 82
Write Out Your Goals and Meal Plan — 85
Shopping List and Stock Pile List — 88
Challenges In Phase 1 — 89
4 Easy Go-To Recipes — 94

PHASE 2: Eliminate	95
Foods to Eliminate	95
Challenges In Phase Two	97
PHASE 3: Refine and Troubleshoot	105
Refine and Adjust	105
Troubleshoot Your Diet	107

Part 3: Recipes

BREAKFAST AND SMOOTHIES	114
Carrot Cake Oat Bowl	115
Easy Balanced Oat Bowl	116
Peanut Butter Chocolate Oats	117
No Bake Energy Bites	118
Easy Oat Waffles	119
Tropical Sunrise Chia Pudding	120
Black Forest Cake Smoothie	121
Easy Berry Breakfast Smoothie	122
High Protein Green Smoothie	123
Immunity Boosting Smoothie	124
Grapefruit Banana Green Smoothie	125
Sweet Potato Green Smoothie	126

SALADS AND SANDWICHES 127

Caprese Pasta Salad 128

Roasted Vegetable Salad (Autumn Edition) 129

3 Salad Dressings 130

Easy Lentil Salad 131

Homemade Hummus 132

Avocado Bagel 134

Greek Pita With Tzatziki Sauce 135

LUNCH AND DINNER RECIPES	136
Mexican Stuffed Sweet Potatoes	138
	138
Creamy Butternut Squash Spaghetti	139
	139
Cauliflower Potato Stew	140
	140
Italian Asparagus Gnocchi	141
	141
Fajita Rice Bowl	142
Easy Black Bean Mushroom Burger	143
Lemon Crema Farfalle	145
Thai Noodle Soup	146
Peanut Sauce Stir Fry	147
Mushroom Stroganoff	148
Curried Chickpeas with Water-Fried Potatoes	149
Creamy Tofu Tomato Linguine	150
Easy Lentil Soup	151
Butternut Ginger Soup (or Sweet Potato)	152
Vegan Sloppy Joe's	153
Roasted Vegetable Sheet Pan (Autumn Version)	154
Bean Ball Marinara	155
Burrito Bowl with Avocado Lime Crema	156
One Pot Zucchini Pasta	157
Sweet Potato Chili	158
Creamy Coconut Potato Stew	159
Taco Elbow Pasta	160

	160
Easy Mashed Potatoes	161
Mushroom Gravy	162
Mushroom Bean Balls With Gravy and Rice	163
Creamy Pinto Bean Potato Soup	164

Part 4: Meal Plans

HIGH PROTEIN MEAL PLAN	166
~2000 Calories | ~123 g Protein | 6 Days	166
WEIGHT LOSS MEAL PLANS	169
MEAL PLAN FOR BEGINNERS	169
~ 1750 Calories | ~72 g Protein | 8 Days | GF Option	169
NO-COOK LUNCH MEAL PLAN	173
~1750 Cal | ~82 g Protein | 8 Days	173
SEASONAL MEAL PLANS & FAMILY MEAL PLANNING	177
SPRING/SUMMER MEAL PLAN	177
~ 1790 Calories | ~67 g Protein | 6 Days	177
FALL/WINTER MEAL PLAN	180
~1700 Cal | ~70 g Protein | 6 Days | 2 Person	180
KID FRIENDLY FAMILY MEAL PLANNING	183
Acknowledgments	187
Resources	188
About The Author	189

INTRODUCTION: My Vegan Story

My name is Lisa Goodwin, author and administrator of 2sharemyjoy.com. I grew up in Germany where I met my American husband. I earned my sport, theology, and teaching degree while in Germany at University of Saarland. Along the way, our family grew and we contemplated making a change.

In 2016 we decided to move from Germany to the United States. After having my first child and moving to the US (fast food everywhere), I gained some weight pretty quickly. So I started a portion control diet and lost 10 pounds. Afterwards, I basically went back to eating the same way I had before and gained back some pounds. Then I realized this diet did not do much for me. Sure, I starved a little and lost weight quickly, but what about my health? The questions began piling up.

Did I get all my nutrients? What foods are really bad? Is there a diet that can help with weight and health?

Along with struggling to keep a healthy weight, I also suffered from chronic gastritis, migraines, and acne. My stomach constantly produced too much acid which caused the stomach lining to be inflamed at all times. If the stomach is inflamed, chances are your arteries, skin, and other organs are inflamed as well. The stomach helps with nutrient absorption and plays a huge role in immune function for your body. So, I was on the lookout to find a diet that would be a part of my lifestyle and that I would just KNOW is healthy for me. My husband and I tried to cut out sugar and also cut back on gluten for a while.

Then we watched vegan documentaries and became interested in trying the vegan diet. These movies spoke to me because of the health benefits from the vegan diet. They spoke to my husband because each one highlighted the negative impacts on local communities created by large scale livestock farming (google CAFOs). While watching documentaries peaked my interest, it was important to me that I do my own research. I figured scientific studies would be where I focused my attention and trust (and yes, I check who performed the study and if they used control/placebo groups). BUT you can find a study on a random page to back up almost any hypothesis you have about healthy eating. So it's important to look at who performed the study, if they used a control group or placebo group, who financed the study (are they neutral), how long the study was conducted, and other factors. If a study was done on a small group, funded by the industry that relates to the health claim of the study, or other factors were not controlled well, you probably should not give much credit to this study. You really have to do your research thoroughly to find truly scientific health claims.

After checking most common vegan myths and reading endless studies and books, the decision to eat a plant based diet was made pretty swiftly. We literally threw out or gave away all non-vegan food and switched our diet within a few days. While that approach is not recommended, it worked for us. As soon as we understood the benefits of a plant based diet and that we simply don't need animal protein, it was much easier to give up cheese, burgers, and steaks.

After 6 months following a vegan diet I had a blood test done and guess how that turned out? All the values you would expect to be low were either average or above average. Here are some examples:

Test	Personal Results	Reference
Potassium	3.6	(3.7-5.4 MEQ/L)
Calcium	9.6	(8.7-19.4 mg/dL)
Total protein	8.1	(6.4-8.3 G/DL)
Sodium	141	(136-147 MEQ/L)
Glucose (1.5 h after eating)	86	(70-99 mg/dL fasting)
Vitamin D	46	(25-80 ng/ml)
Total cholesterol	112	(Desirable <200 mg/dL, under 150 is excellent)
LDL (bad cholesterol)	54	(Desirable <100 mg/dL, 50-70 is considered excellent)
White blood cells	7.1	(4.1-10.2 K/uL)
Red blood count	4.64	(3.8-5.2 M/uL)
Hemoglobin	14.6	(11.9-15.5 G/DL)

My potassium value was 3.6 and on my lab report it stated this is deficient, but some sources say that 3.6 is low but not deficient. Either way, since then I include more potatoes and bananas in my diet. My husband had similar results and no deficiencies (9 months vegan). It's important to mention that his cholesterol tested over 200 a few times in the past (before eating a healthy vegan diet)! Here are his results 9 months in:

Test	Personal Results	Reference
Vitamin D	34	(25-80 ng/ml)
Sodium	138	(136-147 MEQ/L)
Calcium	9.9	(8.4-10.2 mg/dL)
Protein, total	7.8	(6.4-8.3 G/DL)
Total cholesterol	138	(Desirable <200 mg/dL, under 150 is excellent)
LDL (bad cholesterol)	80	(Desirable <100 mg/dL, 50-70 is considered excellent)
Red blood count	5.16	(3.8-5.2 M/uL)
Hemoglobin	15.8	(11.9-15.5 G/DL)

To deepen my education in nutrition I earned my Certificate in Food, Nutrition, and Health (Allegra) through our local college and completed the Vegan Nutritionist Diploma (CPD) from the Centre of Excellence, UK.

Now we feel much better, have more energy and, as an added bonus, we reduced our impact on the environment. Personally, I no longer experience chronic gastritis and I haven't had a migraine in almost one year (compared to once a month). I also believe that my family will experience more long-term health benefits. We started the vegan diet because of the studies and books we read. We stuck to the vegan diet because our real life experience has proven it is much better for our health.

Today, I've made it my passion to teach others how to prepare healthy vegan meals, the benefits of a vegan diet and, more so, I provide the information you need to live healthy and feel amazing, too.

This book will provide you with the information needed to achieve healthy, balanced nutrition and the steps you can take to make necessary changes based on YOUR needs and lifestyle. The goal is not to eat a 100% perfect vegan diet, but to improve your diet week by week and make lifestyle changes that feel natural and have a big impact on your health. No matter what your goal is: budget friendly eating, losing weight, saving more time, balancing a deficiency, reversing a disease, or simply eating more veggies, this book will give you the knowledge, tips, hacks, recipes, and other tools to make it work.

PART 1: VEGAN DIET 101

In Part 1 we will take a deeper look into the vegan diet: The benefits of a plant based diet, making sense of macro nutrients (fat, carbs, protein), how to balance your meals, and how to consume enough micronutrients (vitamins and minerals). You will also learn the foods that are vegan but should be reduced or avoided, all about calories, and how to lose weight or build muscle on a vegan diet.

CHAPTER 1: The Many Ways of Healthy

Search for health advice and you will find information about every food and diet that has ever been tried. If you feel confused about what is healthy, don't worry, you're not alone. We'll work out the best approach to meet your nutritional needs.

First, I want to mention that some foods may be healthy for one person and may not be healthy for another person. For example, some people have allergies or a disease that will cause adverse reactions to certain foods. Someone who just had colon surgery is not supposed to eat high fiber foods even though fiber is very important and healthy to the general population. While a high fiber diet would have helped prevent colon cancer, it is not considered healthy for the person who just went through colon surgery.

Another example: If someone simply can't stick to drinking green smoothies and instead reverts back to eating cookies, the smoothies are not a good health food option for this person. It would be better to find food options with some health benefits that this person can actually stick to, like homemade oat cookies. I want to point out that healthy eating, sometimes referred to as clean eating, comes in stages. There is no black or white. Even on a vegan diet there are plenty of food items that are not healthy, such as vegan cheese or meat substitutes, sugar, certain oils, and margarine. You can always make cleaner, healthier choices so there is a hierarchy of eating habits. You could consider cutting out sodas, but completely cutting out sugars is the healthier option. Additionally, it is healthier to drink a coffee black instead of adding sugar, but if you have been consuming one can of soda per day (33 g sugar), one cup of coffee with one tablespoon of sugar (12 g sugar) is a healthier option.

Another problem that occurs is the misconception of following 'clean recipes' or buying 'health products.' If you have been using natural sweeteners like honey to sweeten your meal or drink your body reacts the same way to the "natural" sugar as it does to processed sugars. Another example is sea food. Fish is one of the most contaminated foods, but if you eat home cooked fish with a large side of vegetables and whole grains instead of a McDonald burger you have made a healthier, or cleaner, choice.

The phrase "healthy eating" is very loose and can mean many things. It is determined by trends, culture, and experience. If you ever find yourself confused about what is healthy, here is a simple thought process: there have been studies, rumors, and conversations about meat being unhealthy and possibly carcinogenic. I have never heard about any negative health effects from vegetables. There has never been confusion about broccoli being healthy or lists of side effects from eating too much broccoli!

Some clear healthy eating habits that most people agree with are: eat more vegetables and less processed foods. From this point forward I would like to help you assess your current eating habits and help you determine the dietary changes that are best for you. These changes will then be healthy for your situation and should fit your lifestyle. I don't want to tell you exactly how to eat. Rather, I want you to take the information and tools I provide so you can transform your eating habits step by step. Please free yourself from perfectionism and know that healthy eating is a process. Continue educating yourself and stay motivated in the process!

CHAPTER 2: Reasons to Leverage the Power of Plants

The vegan diet can reduce weight, risk of type 2 diabetes, high blood pressure, and risk of some cancers. This is great news considering the two leading causes of deaths in the United States are heart disease and cancer[1].

There are many benefits associated with following a plant based diet. Some are backed by science, some are anecdotal. If you start a plant based diet you will reap some benefits. You could also experience multiple improvements to your health and might even see improvements that are not listed below. You can find many small and large scale studies documenting the benefits of a plant based diet to back up health claims. In this chapter I will focus on some of the most convincing studies.

Plant Power #1: Healthy Weight

In 2016, 39.8% of US adults over the age of 20 were obese and 71.6% were overweight or obese[2]. In 1988-1994, 56% of the population was overweight or obese[3]. The numbers and associated health issues caused by being overweight continue to climb. A tool to measure your weight status is called the body mass index (BMI). It is an index that is calculated based on the height and weight of a person. The exact formula is:

$BMI = weight (kg) / [height(m)]^2$ or $BMI = 730 \times weight (lbs) / [height (in)]^2$

This index is grouped into 4 categories of body mass to help determine whether a person is underweight (below 18.5), normal weight (18.5-24.9), overweight (25-29.9), or obese (greater than 30). The BMI calculation can help health care providers assess certain health risks. For example, a normal BMI correlates with the best health related quality of life[4]. Compared to obese men and women between the ages 50 and 75, women who stay within a normal BMI experience 7 extra years without chronic disease and men experience 9 more years without chronic disease[5]. There is a strong positive correlation between BMI and common chronic diseases, meaning the higher the BMI the higher the risk of developing diseases such as type II diabetes and cardiovascular disease[6].

The Adventist Health Study 2 is one of the biggest studies comparing the vegan diet to vegetarian and omnivore diets. 96,000 cohort members were enrolled throughout the United States and Canada between 2002 and 2007. 7.7% of cohort members were vegan, 29.2% lactoovovegetarian, 9.9% pescovegetarian, 5.4% semivegetarian, and 47.7% nonvegetarian (omnivore)[7]. This study is significant because of the large number of participants, the length of the study, and the control groups. The BMI comparison shows that only the vegan diet group averaged a normal BMI, and all other groups averaged in the overweight section.

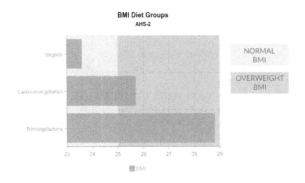

Plant Power #2: Reduced Risk of Type 2 Diabetes

About 9.4% of the US population suffer from type II diabetes[8] and it is the 7th leading cause of death in the US. The Adventist Health Study 2 also found that type 2 diabetes was prevalent in 2.9% of vegans and 7.6% of nonvegetarians, which is a difference of 61%. The study looked at 41,387 participants who did not have diabetes at the beginning of the study. Two years later the diabetes rate occurred in 0.54% of vegans and 2.12% of nonvegetarians. On a large scale it seems like a small difference. But in reality this means 877 people developed diabetes on the nonvegetarian diet, and 223 people developed diabetes on the vegan diet. This is a difference of over 600 people, showing vegans are four times less likely to develop Type 2 diabetes.

Once you have type II diabetes the risk of nerve damage, eye problems, dental, heart and kidney disease, stroke, and foot problems increases[9].

Another review[10] looked at multiple studies: The California studies of Adventists, The Health Food Shoppers' Study, The Oxford Vegetarian Study, and the Heidelberg Vegetarian Study in Germany. This review concluded that vegans average a healthy BMI, have a 78% reduced risk of type 2 diabetes, and a 75% reduced risk of high blood pressure.

Plant Power #3: Reversal and Prevention of Heart Disease

High cholesterol levels increase the risk of stroke and heart disease. Your body makes all the cholesterol it needs and there is no need for any cholesterol intake through diet. The National Research Council recommends a blood cholesterol level under 200 mg/dL but there is evidence that total serum cholesterol levels should be kept below 150 mg/dL[11]. Because vegans don't eat cholesterol, most are naturally within the healthy range. For example, my cholesterol levels were 112 mg/dL when I got my blood test done. My husband got his levels taken before the vegan diet and they were over 200 mg/dL multiple times and never under 170 mg/dL. Nine months into the vegan diet his level is at 138 mg/dL.

Dr. Esselstyn put 18 patients with established coronary disease on a plant based diet (whole food plant based, no oils)[12]. The intervention stopped the progression of the disease and 70% of the patients saw an opening of their clogged arteries. This study was very small with only 18 people, so some view this study with skepticism. However, one particular patient (44 years old) was experiencing acute pain in his left arm, jaw, and chest, which turned out to be a clogged coronary artery. His total cholesterol was 156 mg/dL and LDL was 97 mg/dL. He was put on a whole food plant based diet without any medication and 32 months later the disease was completely reversed. The artery was fully cleared of the blockage!

Plant Power #4: Cancer Prevention

According to the cancer center in Texas[13], 90% of cancer is caused by lifestyle. A healthy diet, the avoidance of alcohol and smoking, and keeping a healthy BMI can potentially cut your cancer risk by 62-82%. Also, avoiding red meat and processed meat can decrease the risk of developing cancer. According to the International Agency for Research on Cancer, processed meat consumption is a group 1 carcinogen (known carcinogen) and red meat is a group 2A carcinogen (probable carcinogen)[14]. Colorectal cancer is the second leading cause of cancer death in the United States. In one study, 1,905 participants[15] were evaluated once they completed the full trial follow-up. The study found that daily bean consumption reduces the chance of developing pre-cancer clusters (for colon cancer) up to 65 percent, a pretty significant number simply by switching your meat with beans. In another study, different cancer cells (from prostate, stomach, breast, and other cancers) were treated with the milk protein casein and the prostate cancer cells rapidly increased in number (enhanced by 134% and 142%)[16]. However, this study was performed in vitro so it's unclear how this would perform in our bodies. On the other side, antioxidants are important to fight off free radicals that cause cancer so it would be very interesting to see what happens if you apply antioxidants to cancer cells. That is exactly what this study[17] did: Different berry extracts (high in antioxidants) were tested for their antiproliferative effectiveness using human cervical cancer and colon cancer cells grown in microtiter plates. The strawberry extract especially slowed cancer cell growth (in vitro).

I could count many more benefits of eating a plant based diet, from reduced migraines and acne to lower risk of arthritis, but studies supporting these findings are smaller and not as representative. Simply put: the vegan diet does not just target one problem like weight loss, heart disease, cancer, or diabetes. Instead, it works for broad spectrum health improvements!

Notes

1. National Center for Health Statistics. (2019). FastStats. Retrieved from https://www.cdc.gov/nchs/fastats/leading-causes-of-death.htm
2. National Center for Health Statistics. (2019, September 4). FastStats. Retrieved from https://www.cdc.gov/nchs/fastats/obesity-overweight.htm
3. CDC. (2019). Retrieved from https://www.cdc.gov/nchs/data/hus/2018/026.pdf
4. Laxy, M., Teuner, C., Holle, R. et al. The association between BMI and health related quality of life in the US population: sex, age, and ethnicity matters. Int J Obes 42, 318–326 (2018)
5. Stenholm, S., Head, J., Aalto, V., Kivimäki, M., Kawachi, I., Zins, M., ... Goldberg, M. (2017). Body mass index as a predictor of healthy and

disease-free life expectancy between ages 50 and 75: a multicohort study. Retrieved from https://www.ncbi.nlm.nih.gov/pmc/articles/PMC5418561/

6. Fontana, L., & Hu, F. B. (2014). Optimal body weight for health and longevity: bridging basic, clinical, and population research. Retrieved from https://www.ncbi.nlm.nih.gov/pmc/articles/PMC4032609/

7. Orlich, M. J. & Fraser, G. E. (2014). Vegetarian diets in the Adventist Health Study 2: a review of initial published findings. Retrieved from https://www.ncbi.nlm.nih.gov/pmc/articles/PMC4144107/

8. Centers for Disease Control and Prevention. (2018). National Diabetes Statistics Report. Retrieved from https://www.cdc.gov/diabetes/data/statistics/statistics-report.html

9. National Institute of Diabetes and Digestive and Kidney Disease. (2016). What is Diabetes? Retrieved from https://www.niddk.nih.gov/health-information/diabetes/overview/what-is-diabetes#problems

10. Fraser, G. E. (2009). Vegetarian diets: what do we know of their effects on common chronic diseases? Retrieved from https://www.ncbi.nlm.nih.gov/pmc/articles/PMC2677008/

11. Esselstyn, C. B. (n.d.). In Cholesterol Lowering, Moderation Kills. Retrieved from http://www.dresselstyn.com/site/study05/

12. Esselstyn, C. B. (2007). Resolving the Coronary Artery Disease Epidemic Through Plant'Based Nutrition. Retrieved from https://onlinelibrary.wiley.com/doi/full/10.1111/j.1520-037X.2001.00538.x

13. Anand, P., Kunnumakara, A. B., Sundaram, C., Harikumar, K. B., Tharakan, S. T., Lai, O. S., ... Sung, B. (2008). Cancer is a Preventable Disease that Requires Major Lifestyle Changes. Retrieved from https://www.ncbi.nlm.nih.gov/pmc/articles/PMC2515569/

14. American Cancer Society. (2019). Known and Probable Human Carcinogens. Retrieved from https://www.cancer.org/cancer/cancer-causes/general-info/known-and-probable-human-carcinogens.html

15. Lanza, E., Hartman, T. J., Albert, P. S., Shields, R., Caan, B., Paskett, E., ... Iber, F. (2006). High Dry Bean Intake and Reduced Risk of Advanced Colorectal Adenoma Recurrence among Participants in the Polyp Prevention Trial. Retrieved from https://www.ncbi.nlm.nih.gov/pmc/articles/PMC1713264/

16. Park, S., Kim, J., Kim, Y., Lee, S. J., Lee, S. D., & Chung, M. K. (2014). A Milk Protein, Casein, as a Proliferation Promoting Factor in Prostate Cancer Cells. Retrieved from https://www.ncbi.nlm.nih.gov/pmc/articles/PMC4166373/

17. McDougall, G. J., Ross, H. A., Ikeji, M., & Steward, D. (2008). Berry Extracts Exert Different Antiproliferative Effects against Cervical and Colon Cancer Cells Grown in Vitro. Retrieved from https://pubs.acs.org/doi/10.1021/jf073469n

CHAPTER 3: Making Sense of Carbs, Protein, and Fat

Carbohydrates, protein, and fat, also called macronutrients, are three big nutrient groups that your food can be divided into. Each macronutrient plays an important role in your diet. A potato contains more carbs than protein or fat, therefore, it would fall into the carbohydrate group. An avocado would fall into the fat group and tofu would fall into the protein group. Some people, especially athletes, believe you have to eat a certain ratio of each group in order to reach specific fitness goals.

However, rather than focusing on percentages, it is better to focus on a variety of whole plant foods. If you do so you automatically eat each macronutrient and no counting is required. Here is an example: Meat contains fat and protein but zero carbs or fiber. Lentils, on the other hand, are high in protein but also contain carbs, fat, and fiber. Lentils contain all macro nutrients plus fiber. As a result, they are considered a whole plant based food. You would not get all your macronutrients when eating meat, whereas by eating plants you would. When eating animal derived food you would have to make sure you don't exceed the recommended saturated fat intake per day. This is not the case when eating whole plant food because unprocessed plant based food is very low in saturated fat.

In this chapter we will make sense of the different foods that are associated with each macronutrient group and also shine some light on fiber consumption. This information is an important foundation for understanding nutrition and finding the right plant foods for your needs.

Carbohydrates

Carbohydrates, or carbs for short, are the body's first energy source. Carbohydrates are made (by the plant) from carbon and water. When we eat the plants and burn the carbohydrates they break back down into water and carbon which then fuels us with energy. Carbohydrates provide energy to your whole body, help the body absorb protein, and are required in the largest amount. There are two forms of carbohydrates: complex and simple.

Complex carbs are surrounded by fiber which causes the food to break down slower. Therefore, it won't spike insulin levels like simple carbs. Instead, it fuels your body with lasting energy.

Simple carbs don't contain any fiber, break down quickly, are refined (stripped of nutrients) or processed, and have similar effects on your blood sugar levels as table sugar. Simple carbs can cause your blood sugar levels to quickly spike and fall. This usually makes individuals feel sluggish, tired, and quick to hunger. Most often these simple carbs are mixed with lots of fat, like in donuts or potato chips. Simple carbs should be avoided, whereas complex carbs are beneficial to your health.

Any carb-heavy food that is processed, refined, lacks fiber, or has multiple ingredients on the label is usually a simple carb. This would include most breads, some cereals, prepackaged snacks and treats, yogurts, and so on. The easiest way to find complex carbs is to focus on whole plant foods: whole oats, beans, vegetables, fruits. Healthy carbs are also high in fiber, sometimes contain water, are not processed, and do not have added ingredients like sugar and oil.

Here's a great example; if you compare the ingredient labels of whole wheat and white pasta, whole wheat pasta contains more fiber per carb than white pasta and some pasta types only contain one ingredient. You can also try chickpea pasta which contains more fiber and protein than white or whole wheat pasta! Bread often contains white wheat, a simple carb, and a long ingredient list. Some breads even contain added sugar and oil. Ezekiel bread usually contains good ingredients and is high in fiber, but tends to be a little on the expensive side.

If you eat plenty of fiber throughout the day and you are a healthy person then the occasional "simple carb" won't hurt. You can read more about this later in the sugar section. Below is an overview of some carbohydrate rich foods for comparison. The more fiber per carbs, the better.

Food	Carbohydrates	Fiber
1 cup white pasta (simple carb)	43 g	2.5 g
1 cup chickpea pasta (complex carb)	38.4 g	9.6 g
1 cup whole wheat pasta (complex carb)	42 g	5.5 g
200 calories white bread (simple carb)	38 g	2.1 g
200 calories whole oats (complex carb)	35.6 g	5.3 g
1.5 cups potato chips (simple carb)	20 g	2 g
Glazed donut (simple carb)	30 g	1 g

Protein

Protein is considered the "building block" of your body and the body's secondary energy source. It is important for your organs, skin, hormones, and muscles. The official daily recommendation of protein is:

- 46 g of protein per day for the average woman
- 56 g of protein per day for the average man

If you are very active or older you might have a higher demand. Proteins are broken down into amino acids and peptides. There are 20 amino acid "building blocks" of protein. Some people worry that they don't get a complete amino profile (equal amounts of all amino acids) while consuming plant based protein. However, eating a variety of plant protein and getting enough calories will complete your amino profile. Complete plant based protein sources include soy, quinoa, hemp, and chia. Here are the best plant based protein sources:

Seeds

- 1 oz hemp seeds (unhulled): 7 g protein, 150 calories
- 1 oz chia seeds: 4.7 g protein, 127.8 calories
- 1 oz pumpkin seeds: 8.5 g protein, 162 calories

Nuts

- Almonds (12 whole, raw): 3.1 g protein, 85 calories
- Walnuts (8 halves, raw): 2.5 g protein, 105 calories

Grains

- 1 cup cooked oats: 6 g protein, 166 calories
- 1 cup cooked buckwheat groats: 5.7 g protein, 154 calories
- 1 cup cooked quinoa: 8.1 g protein, 222 calories
- 1 cup cooked amaranth: 9.4 g protein, 257 calories
- 1 cup cooked brown rice: 5.5 g protein, 248 calories

Legumes

- 1 cup cooked black beans: 15.2 g protein, 227 g calories
- 1 cup cooked lentils: 17.9 g protein, 230 calories
- 1 cup cooked green peas: 8.2 g protein, 124 calories

Vegetables

- 1 cup cooked broccoli: 3.7 g protein, 54 calories
- 1 cup chopped and cooked mushrooms: 3.4 g protein, 43 calories
- 1.25 cup chopped leafy greens: 3 g protein, 25 calories

Soy

- 0.5 block tofu: 14.7 g protein, 126 calories
- 1 cup unsweetened organic and fortified soy milk: 7.8 g protein, 73 calories
- 1 cup cooked soy beans: 31.3 g protein, 295 calories

Fats

Fats are the third macronutrient and are part of a balanced diet. Just like carbs, there are different types of fats that have different effects on your body. Compared to carbohydrates and protein (4 calories per gram), fats contain 9 calories per gram which makes them more calorie dense. Fats maintain healthy skin, support hormone production, and help the body maintain heat. Babies and children especially need fats for brain development. Fats also help absorb fat soluble vitamins (vitamin A, D, E, K). Essential fatty acids are fats that the body acquires from food and can't make on its own.

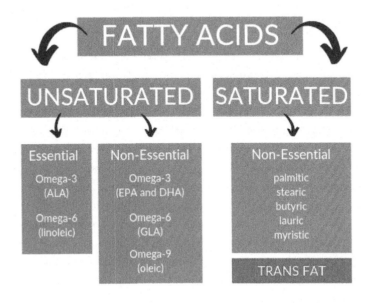

Omega 6 and 3

Omega 6 fatty acids are important for brain health, metabolism, and hair growth. While omega 6 fatty acids are healthy on a balanced diet, they do have an inflammatory effect when consumed too much. Omega 3 fatty acids, on the other hand, have an anti-inflammatory effect. On a typical western diet the omega 6 consumption is too high and the omega 3 consumption is too low. The key is to balance both fats for a healthy diet. The Center for Genetics, Nutrition, and Health[1] found that a ratio of 4/1 was associated with a 70% decrease in total mortality, a ratio of 2-3/1 suppressed inflammation in patients with rheumatoid arthritis, a ratio of 5/1 had a beneficial effect on patients with asthma, but a ratio of 10/1 had adverse consequences. Many processed foods contain low quality oils that increase omega 6. Cutting out fast food and processed food will already clear up most of the inflammation factors. Omega 6 is also found in whole plants like soy beans and walnuts (in a healthy ratio).

On the other hand, you can increase omega 3 easily by adding (ground) flaxseed to your cereal, smoothies, and salads. Walnuts, chia seeds, and hemp seeds are another great source of omega 3. There are actually two types of omega 3 fatty acids: ALA and DHA (+EPA). ALA is found in plants mostly in flaxseed and walnuts and DHA is found in fish and algae. Our bodies can transform ALA to DHA. To transform ALA into the recommended amount of DHA (on a vegan diet) we would need to eat approximately 2 tablespoons of flaxseed per day. You only need to supplement with DHA (algae) if your body can't transform ALA for various health reasons (which is rare). There is also evidence that we might not need as much DHA as previously thought. However, some vegans choose to take DHA algae supplements as a precaution and in an attempt to prevent Alzheimer's disease.

Plant based omega-3 sources (ALA):

- 2 tablespoons flax seed (ground): 1.8 g
- 10 walnut halves: 1.8 g
- 1 tablespoon chia seeds: 1.8 g
- 2 tablespoons unhulled hemp seeds: 1.4 g
- 1 cup natto: 1.3 g
- ½ cup soy beans: 0.5 g
- 1 cup cooked brussel sprouts: 0.4 g
- 1 cup cooked wild rice: 0.2 g

Saturated Fats

Saturated fat raises your cholesterol and increases risk of heart disease and stroke. The American Heart Association (2015) suggests eating no more than 5-6 % of your diet in saturated fat per day. If 9 calories equals 1 gram of fat that means you should eat no more than 13.3 g saturated fat per day on a 2000 calorie diet.

Here is an overview of the saturated fat content for each food item per ½ cup:

- Coconut oil 89.9 g
- Palm oil 53.2 g
- Coconut milk, canned 15 g
- Olive oil 15 g
- Peanut butter 13.3 g
- Cheddar cheese 10.7 g
- Hamburger 3.8 g
- Cocoa powder 3.5 g
- Whole milk 2.3 g
- Black beans 0.1 g

The overview above shows that there is actually a lot of saturated fat in plant based food, most of which is found in processed foods like oils. Therefore, I suggest sticking to whole plant foods as much as possible. If you look at the table above and compare the saturated fat content from olive oil with cow's milk it seems like olive oil contains more saturated fat. This is true if you compare one half of a cup of each liquid. But if you compare serving sizes, the numbers look different. It is more likely to use one teaspoon of olive oil for a salad, which contains 0.6 g saturated fat, and one cup of cow's milk for cereal, which contains 4.6 g saturated fat. With realistic serving sizes, the animal derived foods usually contain more saturated fat.

Trans Fats

The problem with trans fats is that the body releases free radicals while trying to break down stable fats like trans and saturated fats. Free radicals are known to negatively impact DNA, cells, and their compounds, raise levels of bad cholesterol, and cause inflammation in the body.

The more saturated the oil or fat, the more stable it is at room temperature. If you take this process a step further you have trans fats. With the process called 'hydrogenation' we can take liquid oils and turn them solid or semi solid, like margarine. Frying food can also create trans fats. Some trans fats are produced with this process, but there are also naturally occurring trans fats. These are often found in animal food sources that already contain a high amount of saturated fats. Here are some examples of trans fat containing foods:

- 1 bag microwave popcorn 10.3 g
- 1 cup fried potato tots 4.5 g
- ground beef, 1 medium patty: 0.6 g
- 1 cup whole milk: 0.3 g

As you can see, vegan food can even contain trans fat if it is highly processed but unprocessed plant based whole foods are free of all trans fats. See the chart below for lipid profiles of different foods. Walnuts are the healthiest option in this comparison.

150 Calories of:	Whole Milk (1 cup)	Olive Oil (1.2 tbsp)	Walnuts (11 halves)
Omega 3 (g)	0.2	0.1	2
Omega 6 (g)	0.3	1.6	8.5
Saturated fat (g)	4.6	2.2	1.4
Trans fat (g)	0.3	0	0
Cholesterol (mg)	24.4	0	0

Notes

1. Simopoulos, A. P. (2008). The importance of the omega-6/omega-3 fatty acid ratio in cardiovascular disease and other chronic diseases. Retrieved from https://www.ncbi.nlm.nih.gov/pubmed/18408140?dopt=Abstract

CHAPTER 4: Fiber, Pre-, and Probiotics

Fiber

Fiber is found in plant based foods, is necessary for healthy digestion, and can reduce constipation. Fiber can be divided into two categories, soluble and insoluble. Increased fiber intake has been found to lower risk of stroke, obesity, diabetes, coronary heart disease, certain gastrointestinal diseases, and hypertension[1].

If you have been consuming a standard western diet throughout your life, you most likely are not consuming enough fiber. The American Heart Association (2016) suggests eating at least 25 g of fiber per day on a 2,000 calorie diet. Furthermore, they state that dietary fiber can improve blood cholesterol levels and lower the risk of heart disease, stroke, obesity, and even type 2 diabetes. Generally, fiber promotes healthy digestion, it binds toxins, and keeps you full for longer. The good news is that on a plant based diet you most likely eat much more than 25 g of fiber! Every plant food contains fiber, some more, some less. In comparison, animal derived foods contain ZERO fiber. However, if you switch to a plant based diet I suggest introducing more fiber-rich foods slowly and decreasing animal foods slowly. This will give your gut bacteria time to adjust. Otherwise you may experience digestive issues for a few days or even weeks. You will learn how to transition slowly into a fiber rich diet in Part 2 of this book.

Soluble and Insoluble Fiber

Soluble fiber dissolves in water and also absorbs water during the digestion process. The insoluble fiber is the one that makes your stool softer to pass quickly through your intestines. If you are on a vegan diet and passing soft stool multiple times per day, you are eating a lot of insoluble fibers. If your stool gets too thin, try switching to more soluble fiber foods. Most plants contain a part of each type, some are richer in one or the other.

Food higher in soluble fiber are:

- flax seed
- grape juice
- kale
- pears
- oranges
- parsnip
- white pasta
- Brussels sprouts
- and cooked broccoli

Foods higher in insoluble fiber are:

- bran
- dates
- almonds
- lentils
- avocado
- buckwheat
- peanuts
- sunflower seeds
- walnuts
- coconuts
- barley

- beans
- and whole wheat pasta

Too Much Fiber on a Vegan Diet?

Fiber in large amounts, especially a sudden increase of such, can cause discomfort or digestive issues like bloating, diarrhea, gas, cramping, and constipation. On a whole food vegan diet you can easily eat between 60 g to 80 g of fiber per day following a 2000 calorie diet plan. There is not a clear fiber intake limit provided by nutrition authorities. Duke University (2015) states that 70 g fiber a day should not be exceeded. However, cultures like rural China (1980) were eating over 70 g of fiber per day and the rural African diet even consumed up to 120 g of fiber per day and heart disease was almost non-present. Personally, I eat between 60 and 80 g of fiber per day and my gut health is excellent. If you already eat more than 60 g of fiber per day and you don't have any insulin resistance you can enjoy a side of white pasta and white rice instead of whole wheat products.

When to Eat Less Fiber?

Reduce fiber intake if you suffer from Crohn's disease, have had surgery on your intestines, or suffer from bloating or extremely soft stool after months on a vegan diet. Sometimes the bloating can be caused by other issues, like foods allergies or sensitivities to new recipes or spices.

Here are some things to consider if you experience discomfort in your intestines:

#1 Drink more water.

If you consume a lot of soluble fiber, drinking more water can help with digestion.

#2 Take walks/exercise.

Working out and being active provides many health benefits, including better digestion and metabolism.

#3 Eat smaller meals.

Plant based food has a higher volume per calorie. Often times a large amount of plant food is simply too much to process for your gut. Try to eat slowly, chew well, and eat smaller meals.

#4 Reduce fiber intake.

If you are exceeding 70 g of fiber per day and you think this might be the cause of your discomfort, include more low fiber foods such as: white pasta, potatoes, white rice, tofu, vegan cheese, vegan yogurt, etc. However, keep substitutions to a minimum. It is still very important to eat lots of fiber. Try to reduce fiber only a little bit at first and make small changes at a time.

#5 Drink fennel tea.

This tea is a great natural remedy for bloating and it increases hydration. We even used it on our baby (after 2 weeks of age) when he experienced bloating.

#6 Chew well.

If you don't chew your food properly or you eat too fast, you leave more room for air which will end up in your gut. Instead, make sure you chew your food all the way down to a puree before swallowing and see if this reduces bloating. Oftentimes, we don't chew well enough when we don't take time to eat or we eat on the go.

Prebiotic Fiber

Prebiotic fibers stimulate the growth but also the activity of the good gut bacteria (probiotic). Both in combination improve your gut health and your overall health (immune system, skin, etc.,...). Soluble fiber is the only prebiotic that can be metabolized and fermented in your gut.

Probiotics

Probiotics are the good bacteria in your gut. The cells in our digestive system are linked to our immune system. Whenever we experience an unhealthy gut our immune system suffers, as well. This causes our body to become susceptible to other diseases. Poor diet and internal antibiotic use destroy good gut bacteria. Our digestive tract contains about 400 different types of probiotic bacteria and the composition of such depends on your eating habits. For example, if you eat lots of fat, your gut bacteria is adjusted to breaking down fats. The reason why some people get so bloated when they start eating fiber rich foods is because their gut bacteria is not adjusted to breaking down larger amounts of fiber. Therefore, it is important to always ease into a new diet.

As babies we get our set of probiotics during vaginal birth and through drinking breast milk. If a baby did not get probiotics from either and suffers from allergies, asthma, or immune system issues, you can talk to the child's doctor about using probiotics. Later in life, antibiotics surround us everywhere. They might be present in drinking water, antibacterial soaps, liquids, plants, meat, and fish. It's worth noting that 75-80% of antibiotics produced by the pharmaceutical industry are used to treat livestock, inadvertently affecting our health. Some recent research[2] suggests multiple health benefits from increasing probiotic intake: preventing cancer, treating high cholesterol, and improving digestion. Current research is also looking at the use of probiotics to treat diarrhea, urinary tract infections[3], and more. We can find good bacteria in fermented foods like vegan yogurt and cheese, sauerkraut, kombucha, tempeh, miso, kimchi, pickles, apple cider vinegar (with the mother), and supplements.

Prebiotics are not bacteria but they (in the form of nondigestible fiber) help activate the good bacteria. Including a few of these fermented foods with a fiber rich diet can definitely help with overall health. At this point we don't know exact doses and frequency of use. Hence, it is hard to find the right probiotic supplement. If you are researching the best probiotic supplement for yourself, here are some tips: Make sure the label indicates the strain used, the number (CFU) of the live microorganisms, a suggested serving size, health claims of the product, other added ingredients, storage information, and a way to contact the company. Some people balance their gut health by taking probiotic supplements for a couple of weeks. I think the easiest and cheapest way to include larger amounts of probiotics in you diet naturally is by eating sauerkraut once or twice per week. I like to serve sauerkraut with vegan baked beans and oven roasted potato wedges (oil free). Alternatively, you can use steamed edamame seasoned with salt, pepper, and garlic powder.

Notes

1. Anderson JW, et al. (2009). Health benefits of dietary fiber. Retrieved from https://www.ncbi.nlm.nih.gov/pubmed/19335713
2. Kumar, M., Nagpal, R., Kumar, R., Hemalatha, R., Verma, V., Kumar, A., ... Chakraborty, C. (2012). Cholesterol-Lowering Probiotics as Potential Biotherapeutics for Metabolic Diseases. Retrieved from https://www.ncbi.nlm.nih.gov/pmc/articles/PMC3352670/
3. Falagas ME, et al. (2006). Probiotics for prevention of recurrent urinary tract infections in women: a review of the evidence from microbiological and clinical studies. Retrieved from https://www.ncbi.nlm.nih.gov/pubmed/16827601

CHAPTER 5: Mastering Micronutrients

Micronutrients are the nutrients your body needs in smaller amounts to function properly and stay healthy. These are vitamins and minerals. Besides the importance of consuming all your larger food groups (macros: carbs, protein, fat, and fiber) you need to make sure to get all your vitamins and minerals, as well. This is not as complicated as it sounds. In this chapter we will take a look at the Recommended Dietary Allowance (RDA) for vitamins and minerals. These numbers were drawn from the Dietary Guidelines for Americans 2015-2020[1]. I'll also show you the plant based foods rich in each vitamin and mineral. This information can help you with deficiencies and meal planning. Finally, we will take a look at supplementation and phytochemicals. Learning about the nutrients within your food will help pin point the foods you want to add to your diet. It will also help you understand the benefits of eating more plants.

Vitamins

Vitamins can be divided into two categories; fat soluble and water soluble. The fat soluble vitamins, which are vitamins A, D, E, and K, can be stored in the body's fat tissue for a while. The water soluble vitamins (all other vitamins) will be excreted after the body has absorbed the necessary amount. These vitamins have to be consumed frequently.

Vitamin A

Vitamin A is a fat soluble vitamin and a powerful antioxidant. It is important for your immune system, your eyes, your organ function, and for reproduction. Night blindness is one of the earliest signs of a vitamin A deficiency. Low iron levels are also associated with a vitamin A deficiency[2]. Preformed vitamin A (retinol) is only found in animal derived foods and a grown woman would need 2310 IU. However, our bodies can convert carotenoids, found in plant based food, into vitamin A. These can be measured in retinol activity equivalents (RAE). Women need about 700 µg RAE (or 8400 µg beta carotene), and grown men need about 900 µg RAE.

Here are some vitamin A rich plant based foods (hint: make sure you eat orange foods):

- 1 cup sweet potato: 1890 µg RAE
- 1 cup carrots: 1290 µg RAE
- 1 cup cubed butternut squash: 1143 µg RAE
- 1 cup cubed cantaloupe: 270 µg RAE
- 1 cup spinach: 140 µg RAE

Here is a great smoothie recipe that you can drink daily to make sure all your needs are met (for men and women). It contains 908 µg RAE:

- ¼ cup sweet potato (raw)
- 2 cups spinach
- 1 cup almond milk (or other plant milk)
- 1 banana
- 1 tablespoon peanut butter (or more for taste)
- 1 teaspoon ground flax seed

This smoothie recipe also contains: 320 calories, 7.8 g fiber, 48 g carbs, 9.5 g protein, 150 mg magnesium, and 3.6 mg iron.

B-vitamins

B-vitamins B1, B2, B3, B5, B6, B7 and B9 (folate) are usually easy to get from a well-planned vegan diet. Nutritional yeast, brown rice, lentils, asparagus, mushrooms, peas, oats, almonds, and sunflower seeds are high in B-vitamins. Be aware, some medications and consumption of alcohol can decrease your B-vitamin levels. B12 is not obtained from a vegan diet. We will go more into detail below. I will also discuss the B9 (folate) vitamin in more detail as it has more specific functions in your body.

B_{12}

B12 plays an important role in red blood cell production, neurological function, and DNA synthesis[3]. Signs of a B12 deficiency include anemia, fatigue, weakness, constipation, loss of appetite, and weight loss. There are some medications that can lower your B12 levels and, when you get older, your body's ability to absorb B12 weakens. It usually takes a while for a B12 deficiency to be detected, therefore, it is important to include this vitamin in your diet. B12 is mostly found in animal derived foods (except honey). It is made by bacteria living in the soil and animals ingest it by eating grass. Because of common modern agricultural practices, most animals are not grass fed anymore. This leads to decreasing B12 levels in animal derived foods. As a result, some livestock are injected with B12 supplements. There are some vegan foods that are fortified with B12 like soy milk, plant based yogurts, and breakfast cereal. Nutritional yeast is another food high in B vitamins. This is a condiment that most vegans use as a Parmesan cheese substitute. In my opinion, it is safest to supplement with B12 tablets. Personally, I take 2500 mcg once a week on Saturday mornings when I make waffles.

Folates (B9)

Folates help prevent anemia (iron deficiency) and are also important for cell and tissue growth. While folate deficiency is not very common, women who want to get pregnant or are pregnant should focus more on folate intake. A folate deficiency during pregnancy can lead to the birth of infants with neural tube defects. In adults, a deficiency in this B-vitamin can show symptoms such as weakness, fatigue, difficulty concentrating, irritability, or headache[4]. For adults, the RDA is 400 mcg derived from food and for pregnant women it is 600 mcg (food derived). Folic acid differs from folate and is found in supplements.

Here are the plant based foods that are high in folate:

- 1 cup raw beets: 308 mcg
- 0.75 cup cooked lentils 268 mcg
- 1 cup edamame: 241 mcg
- 0.75 cup chickpeas: 216 mcg
- 0.75 cup black beans: 180 mcg
- 0.25 cup peanuts: 87 mcg
- 0.5 papaya: 70 mcg
- 0.5 avocado: 60 mcg
- 1 cup spinach 58 mcg
- 1 cup broccoli: 57 mcg

Most of my recipes contain 0.75 cups of legumes per serving. If you prepare them for lunch and dinner, you already met your daily need of folate.

Vitamin C

Vitamin C is an antioxidant that is typically used to boost immunity.

It also helps with collagen formation, the absorption of non-heme iron, and the metabolism of folic acid[5]. Signs of a vitamin C deficiency can include: Scurvy, fatigue, inflammation of the gums, poor wound healing, and anemia (vitamin C helps with iron absorption)[6]. Adult women should consume a minimum of 75 mg and men should consume 90 mg per day. This is pretty easy considering the table below.

Here are some foods high in vitamin C:

- 1 medium yellow bell pepper: 218.4 mg
- 1 medium red bell pepper: 152 mg
- 1 medium green bell pepper: 95.7 mg
- 1 cup raw broccoli: 81.2 mg
- 1 medium grapefruit: 79.9 mg
- 1 medium orange: 69.7 mg

Vitamin D

Vitamin D is important for healthy bones (calcium absorption), muscle function, and a strong immune system. There are more than 3 million people per year (in the US) with vitamin D deficiency. Weak bones, bone pain, and muscle weakness can indicate low vitamin D levels[7]. You can get vitamin D through sunshine and through food. Vitamin D is naturally occurring in mushrooms and you can find it in fortified products like plant milks, breakfast cereal, and orange juice. The recommended amount for women and men under 70 years old is 600 IU per day (15 mcg). One cup of fortified orange juice contains about 100 IU. You can also get your vitamin D naturally through sunlight exposure. This, however, is controversial because of skin cancer risks. The amount of vitamin D your body produces when exposed to UV light depends on your skin type, where you live, what time of day it is, and season. If you don't want to get your vitamin D from sunlight or through food you can also take a supplement. This might be a good solution during the winter months or if you live in northern locations. Personally, I expose my arms and legs to sunlight for about 10 minutes per day or 3 times per week for 15 minutes. I use sunblock for longer periods outside. During very dark winter months in Maryland I supplement with vitamin D tablets. Vitamin D is fat-soluble so be cautious as excessive intake comes with health risks.

Vitamin K

Vitamin K is a fat-soluble vitamin and it's deficiency is rather rare in adults. Some signs of a deficiency are bleeding problems, hemorrhage, and reduced bone mineralization[8]. Women need about 90 mcg of vitamin K per day and men need 120 mcg. The easiest way to get your daily dose of vitamin K is to drink a smoothie with 1 cup of raw baby spinach.

Here are some plant based foods high in vitamin K:

- 1 cup raw brussel sprouts: 155 mcg
- 1 cup raw spinach (or 1 cup mustard greens): 144 mcg
- 1 cup raw kale: 112 mcg
- 1 cup broccoli raw: 92 mcg

Minerals

The minerals discussed in detail are calcium, potassium, magnesium, iron, zinc, iodine, and selenium. Vegans are more likely to show deficiencies in these minerals while the rest of the minerals, like manganese, copper, and phosphorus, are easier to obtain from food.

Calcium

Calcium is important for your vascular system, muscle function, nerve transmission, intracellular signaling, and hormones[9]. Some of the signs of a calcium deficiency include numbness and tingling in the fingers, muscle cramps, lethargy, poor appetite, and abnormal heart rhythms. Men and women ages 19-50 should consume 1,000 mg calcium per day. Women ages 50+ should increase calcium to 1,200 mg per day.

Here are some high calcium plant based foods:

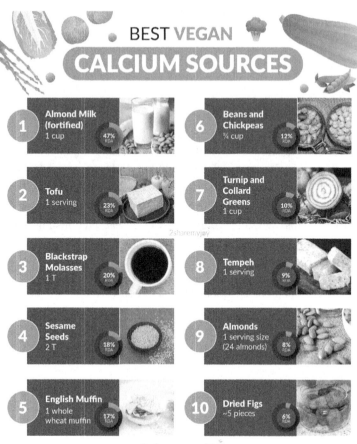

Tahini is simply a paste made out of ground sesame seeds. 2 T of tahini contains 128 mg calcium (~13% RDA). If you have a calcium deficiency you can substitute peanut butter in the recipes with tahini and use it as a dressing, on a sandwich, or in smoothies. I have also noticed that almond milk available in the US is fortified with calcium but overseas it is not. If you live in another country make sure to check your almond milk label. If there is no calcium in it, you have to add calcium rich sources to the recipes in this book. You can do so by adding 1 T blackstrap molasses (as a sweetener) to your oats and 2 T sesame seeds to your smoothies or oats. Eat recipes with tofu often and use sesame butter (tahini) for sauces, dressings, spreads, and smoothies. Some orange juices are fortified with calcium, as well. If you drink orange juice, get the one with added calcium. On the other hand, if you skip juices because of the sugar content, use the whole foods mentioned above to boost calcium intake.

Iron

Iron is important for the production of red blood cells, muscle metabolism, neurological development, cellular functioning, and hormones. A deficiency in this mineral can cause gut issues, anemia, weakness, fatigue, and difficulty concentrating[10]. The iron RDA for women ages 19-50 is 18 mg per day. Adult males and women over 50 should consume 8 mg per day. There is a difference between the iron found in animals and the iron found in plants. Heme iron, foundin animals, is better absorbed but the body can't rid excess heme iron easily. If it is over-consumed, animal derived heme can cause inflammation. Non-heme iron is found in plants (and small amounts in animals) and you might have to eat a bit more of it or pair it with vitamin C rich foods for better absorption. Your body is able to shed excess non-heme iron and balance out iron storages. There is no scientific evidence to support the claim that vegans are iron deficient. You can get healthy iron levels from a balanced plant based diet.

Here are some iron rich foods:

- 1 cup cooked soybeans: 8.8 mg
- 1 cup cooked lentils: 6.6 mg
- 1 cup cooked amaranth: 5.3 mg
- 1 cup cooked chickpeas: 4.7 mg
- 1 cup boiled potato with skin 4.4 mg
- 1 cup cooked black beans: 4.1 mg

- 1 cup cooked oats: 3.4 mg
- 2 tablespoon hemp seed (unhulled): 2.8 mg
- ¼ cup raw cashews: 2.2 mg
- ½ cup dried apricots: 1.7 mg
- 1 tablespoon tahini 1.4 mg
- 1 cup raw brussel sprouts: 1.2 mg
- 24 almonds, raw: 1.1 mg

The following is a high iron 1700 calorie meal plan example (mg of iron):

Breakfast: 1 cup oats (3.4 mg), 1 cup berries (0.7 mg), 1 tablespoon hemp seeds (1.4 mg), 10 almonds (0.5 mg).

Lunch: 1 cup boiled potato with skin (4.4 mg), ¾ cup black beans (3 mg), 1 cup broccoli (0.7 mg). Snack: ½ cup dried apricots (1.7 mg).

Dinner: 1.5 servings of the sweet potato chili (9.2 mg).

Total iron: 25.1 mg

Magnesium

Magnesium is important for healthy nerve and muscle functions, production of energy, and regulation of blood pressure and blood glucose. Common signs of a magnesium deficiency include twitching and cramping muscles, loss of appetite or nausea, fatigue, and weakness[11]. The vegan diet is very rich in magnesium. The recommended magnesium intake for women ages 19-30 years is 310 mg and ages 31-50+ is 320 mg magnesium per day. Men ages 19-30 years need 400 and ages 31-50+ years need 420 mg magnesium per day.

Here are some plant based magnesium sources:

- 1 cup cooked quinoa: 118 mg
- 1 cup oats: 111 mg
- ¼ cup cashews: 94 mg
- 1 cup cooked black beans: 91 mg
- 1 cup potato with skin: 80 mg
- 1 cup cooked chickpeas: 78 mg
- ¼ cup raw peanuts: 61 mg
- 2 cups spinach: 50 mg
- 10 almonds: 33 mg
- 1 banana: 32 mg
- ½ avocado: 20 mg

By eating a variety of plant foods during the day, it is very easy to get the necessary amount of magnesium in your diet.

Potassium

Potassium is required for normal cell function. A deficiency can cause increased blood pressure, kidney stones, and muscle weakness[12]. All adult men and women should consume 4700 mg of potassium per day.

Below is an overview of high potassium plant based foods:

- 1 medium potato with skin: 1128 mg
- 1 cup cooked northern beans: 993 mg
- 1/2 cup dried apricots: 755 mg
- 1 cup cooked lentils: 730 mg
- 1 cup cooked edamame: 675 mg
- 1 cup cooked black beans: 670 mg
- 1 cup cubed butternut squash: 580 mg
- 1 cup cooked chickpeas: 477 mg
- 1 cup orange juice: 443
- 1 banana: 422 mg

- 1 medium cooked sweet potato: 350 mg

It's easy to meet your potassium intake needs, simply eat potatoes on a regular basis and add plenty of legumes to your meals.

Iodine

Iodine deficiency can lead to an enlargement of the thyroid gland and mental developmental problems in children. Iodine is found mostly in soil but some areas have low iodine levels in their soil. Therefore, fruits and vegetables grown in these areas are low in iodine as well. The recommended daily allowance for adults is 150 mcg per day[13]. Iodized salt contains 71 mcg per 1/4 teaspoon. If you use iodized salt for the recipes (1 teaspoon per recipe that serves 4) and you eat 2 servings per day, you would almost meet your daily need. But be careful there is a daily limit on sodium intake. You can read more about salt in the vegan troublemaker chapter. There is also a limit to iodine intake. Consuming more than 1,100 mcg of iodine per day may cause thyroid dysfunction[14]. To increase iodine intake in other ways, sprinkle some seaweed like kelp or nori over salads and soups. If you are not sure about iodine levels you can talk to your health care provider, or refer to the "WHO Global Database on Iodine Deficiency"[15].

Zinc

Zinc is very important for a healthy immune system. All adult females should consume 8 mg and adult men 11 mg of zinc per day. Vegans and vegetarians might need up to 50% more zinc per day[16]. It is a good idea for females to eat 11-12 mg of plant based zinc and for men to eat between 15 to 16.5 mg zinc per day. Signs of a zinc deficiency can show through a weak immune system and loss of appetite.

Foods high in zinc include:

- 3 tbsp hulled hemp seed: 3 mg
- 1 cup oats: 2.9 mg
- 1 cup boiled chickpeas: 2.5 mg
- 1 cup cooked lentils: 2.5 mg
- 1 cup cooked quinoa: 2 mg
- 1 cup cooked black beans: 1.8 mg
- ¼ cup cashews: 1.7 mg
- 3 tbsp pumpkin seeds: 1.7 mg
- 1 cup cooked brown rice: 1.4 mg
- ¼ cup peanuts: 1.2 mg
- ¼ cup chopped almonds: 1 mg

A high zinc meal plan would look like this:

- Breakfast: 1 cup oats, 1 cup almond milk, 2 T hemp seed, 2 T peptitas (pumpkin seeds), 1 cup berries (5.6 mg zinc)
- Lunch: 1 cup chickpeas cooked in BBQ sauce, 2 tomatoes + 1/2 avocado seasoned with salt and pepper (3.5 mg zinc)
- Dinner: 2 servings of the mushroom stroganoff (8.7 mg zinc)

All in all this meal plan contains almost 2200 calories, 106 g protein, and 17.8 g zinc. It even contains more than your RDA of all other minerals.

Selenium

Selenium acts like an antioxidant and is important for many

functions in your body. It plays a role in reproduction, thyroid hormone metabolism, and DNA synthesis.[17] Every adult needs only a small amount of 55 mcg per day. The ultimate plant based selenium source is the Brazil nut. One Brazil nut contains 90 mcg and covers your daily need of selenium. Other sources are brown rice (1 cup = 11 mcg) and sunflower seeds (3 tbsp = 14 mcg). Other plant based foods contain small traces as well, but I suggest always adding 1 Brazil nut a day to your oats, smoothies, or snacks. But be careful! You can also overdo it with selenium. Make sure you don't eat too many Brazil nuts. One a day is enough.

Supplements on a vegan diet

It is always better to get adequate nutrition from the food you eat rather than pills or tablets. With that being said, supplements may be a necessary part of your life. If you are severely deficient in certain vitamins or minerals you might have to supplement for a while. But if you think a multivitamin a day will keep you healthy, you are wrong. The absorption of a compressed vitamin is questionable and you could potentially consume an unhealthy amount of certain vitamins and minerals. For example, studies have found that too much calcium from supplements raise the risk of cancer death[18] but higher calcium intake from foods does not have this effect. When consuming a multivitamin you could reach your daily intake for a certain vitamin but overdo another, so be cautious when taking this approach.

If you already know what deficiencies you have, talk to your doctor about supplements. Even better, find whole plant foods that are rich in the necessary vitamin or mineral and add them more regularly to your diet. You might want to eat a little more of said nutrient than the recommended amount in the beginning to refill your stores. After a while a blood test will tell if your levels are back to normal.

There are many more possible side effects when taking multivitamins. Some people think multivitamins are healthy, boost your immune system, or cover all your nutritional needs. But you run the risk of relying only on the supplement for health. This will cause you to become less motivated to eat actual fruits and vegetables. As a result, you won't develop a healthy lifestyle or habit change. What most multivitamins don't provide are fiber, probiotics, omega-3, and phytochemicals. If you are consuming a multivitamin and are still eating an inflammatory diet, which contains too much saturated fat, sugar, oil, and salt, you are not achieving great health. However, in rare situations, such as pregnancy or deficiencies, certain supplements are necessary. Typical supplements for a vegan diet include vitamin B12, vitamin D, and omega-3 (DHA). You can find out more about each nutrient in their specific section of this book. When it comes to supplements, always consult with your healthcare provider.

Phytochemicals

While micronutrients are essential to health, phytochemicals, the secondary metabolites and powerful molecules in plants, have become more prominent in the studies of cancer prevention and treatment, neurodegenerative diseases, metabolic disease, and restoration of damaged cells[19]. Plants are filled with phytochemicals and a variety of different fruits and vegetables help you obtain these highly beneficial molecules. These nutrients are not found in supplements either.

Phytochemicals also determine the color and flavor of the plant. For example, the phytochemical carotenoid is responsible for the bright red, yellow, and orange color. There are thousands of phytochemicals and scientists are still researching all of their benefits. According to the American Institute for Cancer Research[20], phytochemicals can

- Stimulate the immune system
- Block substances we eat, drink, and breathe from becoming carcinogens
- Reduce the kind of inflammation that makes cancer growth more likely
- Prevent DNA damage and help with DNA repair
- Reduce the kind of oxidative damage to cells that can spark cancer
- Slow the growth rate of cancer cells
- Trigger damaged cells to commit suicide before they can reproduce
- Help to regulate hormones

Here are some of the common phytochemicals, their benefits, and the foods containing them:

Flavonoids are the biggest group of phytochemicals that contain thousands of its type. Flavonoids are found in fruits, vegetables, grains, roots, tea, and wine. They are great anti-oxidants that help fight diseases like cancer, Alzheimer's disease, atherosclerosis, and inflammation[21].

One type of flavonoids is found in soy products that mimic the action of estrogen, therefore, they are called phyto-estrogen. Some people are worried about the use of soy products due to their estrogenic effects. But phyto-estrogens in soy based food actually dock onto the estrogen receptors while prohibiting the actual estrogen from getting in. These phyto-estrogens might work to prevent breast cancer[22]. To increase flavenoids you can make your oats with soy milk, use edamame beans as a side, or eat tofu. Check out the creamy butternut squash spaghetti, lemon crema farfalle, and creamy tofu tomato linguine for added tofu.

Catechins belong to the group of phytonutrients called flavanols. The catechin EGCG (epigallocatechin-3-gallate) is found in the tea plant camellia sinensis. Teas like green tea, black tea, white tea, and oolong tea are derived from this plant. Some of the health benefits of EGCG include improved weight, improved cardiovascular function, and cancer and diabetes prevention[23].

Carotenoids are mostly found in green leafy vegetables and colored fruits like kiwi, tomatoes, and carrots. Carotenoids are anti-oxidants with the power to decrease the risk of cancers and eye disease[24]. You can increase the bioavailability of this phytochemical by adding a healthy fat with its consumption or by blending them to break down the cell walls of the plant[25]. Check out the green smoothies in the recipe section!

Sulphur-containing compounds are found in garlic and cruciferous vegetables like cauliflower and broccoli. These possess anticarcinogenic properties[26]. You can find many recipes containing cruciferous vegetables in this book. Try riced cauliflower and mix it with any rice dish, soup, stew, or pasta sauce.

Reservatrol is another powerful anti-oxidant that is mostly found in grapes but can also be found in berries and red wine. It can fight chronic disease such as inflammation and tumors. It can also slow down or prevent cognitive deterioration[27]. Other research found that grapes help maintain heart health, protect against aging associated diseases and some cancers. And it's worth mentioning that eating whole grapes is a safer choice for health compared to wine and grape juice[28].

Notes

1. Office of Disease Prevention and Health Promotion. (2019). Dietary Guidelines. Retrieved from https://health.gov/dietaryguidelines/
2. National Institutes of Health. (2019). Vitamin A. Retrieved from https://ods.od.nih.gov/factsheets/VitaminA-HealthProfessional/
3. National Institutes of Health. (2019). Vitamin B12. Retrieved from https://ods.od.nih.gov/factsheets/VitaminB12-HealthProfessional/

4. National Institutes of Health. (2019). Folate. Retrieved from https://ods.od.nih.gov/factsheets/Folate-HealthProfessional/
5. Gershoff, S. N. (1993). Vitamin C (Ascorbic Acid): New Roles, New Requirements? Retrieved from https://academic.oup.com/nutritionreviews/article-abstract/51/11/313/1843513
6. National Institutes of Health. (2019). Vitamin C. Retrieved from https://ods.od.nih.gov/factsheets/VitaminC-HealthProfessional/
7. National Institutes of Health. (2019). Vitamin D. Retrieved from https://ods.od.nih.gov/factsheets/VitaminD-HealthProfessional/
8. National Institutes of Health. (2019). Vitamin K. Retrieved from https://ods.od.nih.gov/factsheets/vitaminK-HealthProfessional/
9. National Institutes of Health. (2019). Calcium. Retrieved from https://ods.od.nih.gov/factsheets/Calcium-HealthProfessional/
10. National Institutes of Health. (2019). Iron. Retrieved from https://ods.od.nih.gov/factsheets/Iron-HealthProfessional/
11. National Institutes of Health. (2019). Magnesium. Retrieved from https://ods.od.nih.gov/factsheets/Magnesium-HealthProfessional/
12. National Institutes of Health. (2019). Potassium. Retrieved from https://ods.od.nih.gov/factsheets/Potassium-HealthProfessional/
13. National Institutes of Health. (2019). Iodine. Retrieved from https://ods.od.nih.gov/factsheets/Iodine-HealthProfessional/
14. American Thyroid Association. (2013). ATA Statement on the Potential Risks of Excess Iodine Ingestion and Exposure. Retrieved from https://www.thyroid.org/ata-statement-on-the-potential-risks-of-excess-iodine-ingestion-and-exposure/
15. https://www.who.int/vmnis/iodine/en/
16. National Institute of Health. (2019). Zinc. Retrieved from https://ods.od.nih.gov/factsheets/Zinc-HealthProfessional/
17. National Institute of Health. (2019). Selenium. Retrieved from https://ods.od.nih.gov/factsheets/Selenium-HealthProfessional/
18. Chen, F., Du, M., Blumberg, J. B., Ho Chui, K. K., Ruan, M., Rogers, G., ... Shan, Z. (2019). Dietary Supplement Use, Nutrient Intake, and Mortality Among U.S. Adults. Retrieved from https://annals.org/aim/article-abstract/2730525/association-among-dietary-supplement-use-nutrient-intake-mortality-among-u
19. Budisan, L., Gulei, D., Zanoaga, O. M., Irimie, A. I., Chira, S., Braicu, C., ... Gherman, C. D. (2017). Dietary Intervention by Phytochemicals and Their Role in Modulating Coding and Non-Coding Genes in Cancer. Retrieved from https://www.ncbi.nlm.nih.gov/pmc/articles/PMC5486001/
20. American Institute for Cancer Research. (2019). Phytochemicals: The Cancer Fighters in Your Foods. Retrieved from https://www.aicr.org/reduce-your-cancer-risk/diet/elements_phytochemicals.html
21. Panche, A. N., Diwan, A. D., & Chandra, S. A. (2016). Flavonoids: an overview. Retrieved from https://www.ncbi.nlm.nih.gov/pmc/

articles/PMC5465813/
22. Breastcancer.org. (2013). Foods Containing Phytochemicals. Retrieved from https://www.breastcancer.org/tips/nutrition/reduce_risk/foods/phytochem
23. Isemura, M. (2019). Catechin in Human Health and Disease. Retrieved from https://www.ncbi.nlm.nih.gov/pmc/articles/PMC6384718/
24. Johnson, E. J. (2002). The role of carotenoids in human health. Retrieved from https://www.ncbi.nlm.nih.gov/pubmed/12134711
25. Hammond, B. R., & Renzi, L. M. (2013). Carotenoids. Retrieved from https://www.ncbi.nlm.nih.gov/pmc/articles/PMC3941826/
26. Stoewsand, G. S. (1995). Bioactive organosulfur phytochemicals in Brassica oleracea vegetables--a review. Retrieved from https://www.ncbi.nlm.nih.gov/pubmed/7797181
27. Ramírez-Garza, S. L., Laveriano-Santos, E. P., Marhuenda-Muñoz, M., Storniolo, C. E., Tresserra-Rimbau, E., Vallverdú-Queralt,, A., & Lamuela-Raventós, R. M. (2018). Health Effects of Resveratrol: Results from Human Intervention Trials. Retrieved from https://www.ncbi.nlm.nih.gov/pmc/articles/PMC6317057/
28. Singh, C. K., Liu, X., & Ahmad, N. (2016). Resveratrol, in its natural combination in whole grape, for health promotion and disease management. Retrieved from https://www.ncbi.nlm.nih.gov/pmc/articles/PMC4553113/

CHAPTER 6: Balancing your Meals

As I mentioned in a previous chapter, there is no need to count macronutrients as long as you stick to a variety of whole plant foods. However, it is worth taking a look at the hierarchy of different food groups also called the food pyramid. The food group that is more nutrient dense should be included in your diet more often than the least nutrient dense food group. This is important and can help you avoid nutrient deficiencies. In this chapter we will focus on nutrient dense foods, the vegan food pyramid, and how to easily create balanced meals. With these essentials you will experience greater success on the vegan diet.

Nutrient Density

Vegetables have the highest nutrient density, meaning they contain more nutrients per calorie. This also means you get to eat more while consuming less calories compared to all other foods. In the table below, you will see a comparison of vegetables, legumes, and healthy fats per 110 calories.

110 Calories	Broccoli (vegetable)	Black Beans (plant protein)	Avocado (healthy fat)	Chicken (animal protein)
Volume	3.7 cups	0.45 cup	0.3 cup	0.25 cup
Carbohydrates (g)	22	20.2	5.9	0
Fiber (g)	8.8	8.1	4.6	0
Fat (g)	1.2	0.5	10.5	2.8
Protein (g)	9.5	6.4	1.3	19
Vitamin C (mg/RDA %)	300 (400%)	0.7 (1%)	6 (8%)	0
Calcium (mg/RDA %)	158 (16%)	53 (5%)	8.8 (1%)	9.2 (1%)
Iron (mg/RDA %)	2.5 (14%)	1.8 (10%)	0.4 (2%)	0.7 (4%)
Zinc (mg/RDA %)	1.4 (14%)	0.8 (8%)	0.5 (5%)	0.8 (8%)

As you can see, the vegetables contain more nutrients per calorie. For the fun of it, let's compare the caloric intake and nutrient density of broccoli vs. chicken. As a matter of fact, you would consume 1800 calories, 154 g of plant based protein, and you would exceed the RDA of all vitamins and minerals when you eat 60 cups of broccoli. On the contrary, you would consume 1900 calories, 340 g protein, no carbs, no fiber, and you would be deficient in B1, folate, vitamins A, C, D, E, and K, calcium, copper, iron, and magnesium when you eat only 4.5 cups of chicken. This shows that meat is much less nutrient dense. You would eat a much lower volume of chicken, exceed the calories of broccoli, and would not consume all the nutrients your body needs.

Getting back to veggies, it's obviously not going to be a great day if you attempt to eat 60 cups of broccoli. That's where the other food groups come in. To make this super easy for daily use I have created the vegan food pyramid and an easy guide on how to prepare your plate. This will help reduce the stress of counting any macros while preparing your lunch and dinner meals.

Balancing Your Meals

It is important to eat lots of fruits and vegetables. In the second step, focus on adding legumes to your meals. I generally recommend adding at least 3/4 cup of legumes to each lunch and dinner. Sometimes I add them to my smoothies. Of course, don't miss the healthy grains. While some grains are less nutrient dense than legumes, they still have their place in your diet.

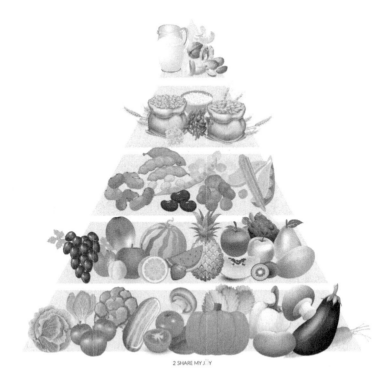

The last food group contains healthy fats and plant based milk. All other food groups in the food pyramid belong to carbohydrate rich or protein rich foods. Nuts and seeds belong to the fat group. Fats contain more calories per gram than carbs and protein. Therefore, the rule of volume eating does not necessarily apply. While whole food plant based fat sources are more nutrient dense than oils, they contain more calories compared to vegetables and smaller amounts are necessary. Fats are an important part of a healthy diet. You can include nuts and seeds with your smoothies and oatmeal, make dressings and sauces out of cashews and avocados, or simply eat nuts as a snack. On the other hand, if you want to gain weight, fat sources like almonds, peanuts, cashews, and walnuts can help increase calories quickly without adding more volume to your plate.

The foods that are not whole foods and are not a part of this food pyramid include sugar, oil, and everything processed. Oil, for example, is not nutrient dense. Because oil lacks nutrients, it is better to use whole plants as a source of fat. You can read more about oils in chapter 7. The foods that are a part of the food pyramid but are somewhat processed include nut butters and plant based milk alternatives. Nut butters are ground whole nuts which can be considered processed, yet they are made of a whole plant food. Nothing is added or stripped. Just be sure to read the food label and avoid added hydrogenated oils and sugar. Almond milk is filtered almond water or watered down almond extract. Although this can be considered processed, only water is added to a whole food. There are no health benefits related to almond milk unless it is fortified with vitamins and minerals, but it can be a great alternative to use for your oats or other recipes. Almond milk contains one third of the calories compared to dairy milk. To ensure you are not consuming an unhealthy product, buy only unsweetened plant milk.

You also won't find any vegan fast food in this pyramid. A vegan junk food diet might save animals, but it is still bad for your health. Vegan junk food like cookies, ice cream, vegan cheese, and vegan meat substitutes are not nutritionally sound and will not fuel your body. Consuming too much of these foods can also lead to nutrient deficiencies. Usually, vegan junk food is refined and stripped of fiber and minerals. Furthermore, junk foods typically contain salt, sugar, and cheap oils. Tip: If you decide to make vegan nuggets on occasion, add 2 cups of steamed broccoli as a side to make your meal a bit healthier.

Breakfast

Oats are a great base for a healthy breakfast. They provide energy, minerals, and fiber. You can create so many different breakfast recipes using oats. To make a balanced breakfast I generally use plant milk and top my oats with lots of fruits, nuts, and seeds. For your convenience, I have provided oat bowl and waffle recipes in this book.

Smoothies and Snacks

Smoothies are a great way to add more veggies, especially dark leafy greens, to your diet. Using the right fruits, you won't even taste them. Always add chia, flax, or hemp seed to your smoothies for added omega-3 and healthy fat. You can add other nuts if you have a good blender. Also, try creating a snack plate with a variety of vegetables, avocado dip, hummus, or nuts.

Lunch and Dinner

An easy way to translate this food pyramid to your lunch and dinner plate is to fill one half with vegetables, one quarter with legumes, and one quarter with a starch. Or: 2 cups vegetables, 3/4 cup legumes, and 3/4 cup starches. If I use broccoli, black beans, and rice for this example, I get about 500 calories and 19 g plant based protein. Depending on your caloric need you can increase these suggestions.

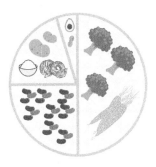

For a salad you can pick 2 cups of dark leafy greens, 2 cups mixed veggies, 1/2 cup starch (quinoa, sweet potato), and 3/4 cup lentils, chickpeas, or beans. Top your salad with an oil free dressing. You can always add healthy fats to these meals: choose avocado, use cashew or tahini dressings, or sprinkle with hemp seeds. This salad is more filling than an iceberg salad with a few slices of cucumber. The legumes and starches add important protein and fiber to your meal and give you lasting energy. All of the recipes in this book are created with the vegan food pyramid in mind.

If you eat mostly white rice for dinner with only a few added vegetables, you are missing out on important nutrients. You can use the same meal but shift your ratios: Add mostly vegetables (2 cups) and a protein source like tofu, edamame, or other legumes. Then sprinkle some sesame seeds over your meal as the fat source. The same goes for salads: Include lots of dark leafy greens, chopped veggies, chickpeas or lentils, and a homemade dressing instead of simple iceberg lettuce with a few tomatoes and store bought dressing. You can even add some cooked quinoa for some healthy whole grains. If the salad doesn't fill you, increase the protein content or simply eat a larger portion.

CHAPTER 7: The 6 Hidden Troublemakers

There are some foods that are not animal derived yet they can be troublesome to your health. Often these foods are hidden, especially in processed foods, and not easily detectable. In this chapter we will talk about the possible dangers of sugar, oil, salt, pesticides, additives, and plastic. We'll also cover healthier options.

Troublemaker #1: Sugar

Sugar is a refined food that doesn't contain any fiber, protein, vitamins, or minerals. It is stripped of everything that is good for your body and can therefore cause damage. Sugar causes inflammation, hormone imbalance, acne, and can lead to a weakened immune system. High sugar consumption raises the risk of heart disease, diabetes, and cancer. Your skin might even age faster. Sugar also has addictive properties. In today's societies, most of us consume too much sugar. It is generally recommended that men eat no more than 37 grams of sugar per day, and women 25 g^1. Food for thought, one soda usually puts you over this limit! Sugar has many sneaky names. Sometimes it is hard to determine whether your food contains added sugar or not. There is a difference between natural sugar found in fruits and vegetables and refined added sugar. Don't be afraid of the sugar found in whole plants. If the food is processed and not a whole plant food, be more cautious. We'll discuss the best approach to understanding which sugar you're consuming later in this chapter.

Do I have to cut out sugar completely?

It is a good idea to limit sugar consumption to the recommended daily amount of 25 g. Depending on your health situation you might want to reduce sugar intake even more. If you are a healthy person and you eat plenty of whole plant foods all day, a little added sugar shouldn't harm you. My personal goal is to stay under 10 g per day. On rare occasions I indulge a little more.

What about sugar substitutes?

Sugar substitutes include artificial sweeteners and natural sweeteners (zero calories). Stevia is a zero calorie natural sweetener and is probably the safest option at this point. I would stay away from all artificial sweeteners. The list of side effects that are linked to artificial sweeteners is not worth the risk in my opinion. Stevia leaves can have a strange after taste, so you might have to get used to the change in taste. Honey (not vegan) and maple syrup are natural sweeteners but cause similar effects on your body as sugar. Compared to sugar, some natural sweeteners contain minerals but not enough to make them an essential health food. Another great natural sweetener (not zero calorie) is date sugar. This is basically dried and ground dates. A downside of this alternative is that they don't dissolve very well. Therefore, they are best used in smoothies, oat bowls, or baking recipes (anything that gets mixed or blended). They would not be a good sweetener for coffee. Date sugar is a whole food dried and ground, so it still contains some fiber. If you don't have any sugar related health problems such as diabetes you can simply work on reducing sugar without finding a substitute. I don't like Stevia and I don't have sugar related health issues so I'm okay with keeping sugar in my diet, just in reduced amounts.

How to reduce or cut out sugar successfully?

Before you begin reducing sugar, it is a good idea to learn how to read labels. There are many names for sugar that you should be aware of. There is also a difference between added sugar and naturally occurring sugar. When it comes to sugar cravings, know that this is just a habit that you have formed over time. Your body is trained to want the same thing over and over. Your first step would be to identify the situation causing you to reach for the sugary foods. Are you drinking the soda for caffeine, as a refreshment, or for energy? Are you grabbing the doughnut after a long day at work? This analysis is so important because once you realize why and when you do these things you can find an alternative that still fits your lifestyle. Below are all the hacks on how to reduce your sugar intake. I want you to start with the easiest one. If you master that one, try the next step. If you struggle just take a step back. It takes time to form new habits. Always make small adjustments to your diet until they become a lifestyle. Then move on to the next adjustment. You decide what your end goal will be. You can try reducing your sugar intake to 25 g per day, 10 g per day, or 25 g per week. This is up to you.

Here are some helpful tips to reduce your sugar intake:

#1 Know how to read labels

There are a few things you should know about reading food labels to detect added sugar. As I mentioned before, there is a difference between natural sugar and added sugar. If you see sugar listed under "ingredients" then you know the sugar is added. If the sugar is ONLY listed in the nutrition facts box and not in the ingredient list then it is natural sugar. You'll notice in the label below there is a line that states "Incl. 0g Added Sugars." Many labels provide this added information for your benefit, but be careful because it is not always provided. Most products that contain natural sugar also contain fiber. You can find the fiber content on your label under total carbs just above total sugars. Be sure to read the ingredients list for a more complete understanding.

Amount per serving	
Calories	**190**
	% DV*
Total Fat 16g	**20%**
Sat Fat 3g	**14%**
Trans Fat 0g	
Cholest. 0mg	**0%**
Sodium 110mg	**5%**
Total Carb. 7g	**2%**
Fiber 3g	**10%**
Total Sugars 2g	
Incl. 0g Added Sugars	**0%**
Protein 8g	**8%**

Here are other names for sugars and sweeteners that you can find within ingredient lists:

- Coconut Palm Sugar
- Corn Syrup
- Dextrin
- Dextrose
- Fructose
- Fruit Juice
- Glucose
- High Fructose Corn Syrup
- Honey
- Lactose
- Molasses
- Palm Sugar
- Saccharose
- Sucrose

- Syrup

#2 Make small adjustments

A consistent and successful transition is made through small adjustments. Count all the added sugar you consume per day and decide which is easiest to cut out or reduce. Let's say you eat a doughnut for breakfast with a coffee that contains 4 teaspoons of sugar. This exceeds the daily recommended amount of sugar for your breakfast. Now you can start reducing your coffee sugar to 3 teaspoons for a few days until it becomes easy. Once you're comfortable go ahead and reduce sugar to 2 teaspoons. The reduction method is much easier than cutting sugar out all at once. If you bring yourself to drinking coffee without sugar, or even very minimal, you can move onto eating half the doughnut and add some sweet fruits on the side. This activity is all about reducing unhealthy choices and replacing with healthy choices step by step.

#3 Start with the smallest obstacle

Tackling the smallest obstacle makes it easier to reduce sugar successfully. From the list of added sugar that you have been consuming, see which one you believe you could live without. You might find it's easy to ditch right away. From there, you want to work your way up to the largest obstacle. Once you have reduced sugar intake, your confidence, taste, and cravings change naturally. Hence, your biggest obstacle will not seem as daunting. And if you are a healthy person there is no harm in keeping some sugar in your diet. If you simply can't ditch your favorite candy bar but you have removed all other added sugar sources, enjoy one candy bar every once in a while. One day you might not crave the same snacks anymore.

#4 Curb cravings naturally

Like I mentioned above, if you focus on sugar reduction while adding more whole foods to your diet your sugar cravings will be reduced naturally. Eating a balanced meal (grains, fats, vitamins, minerals, fiber, protein) WILL help you feel satisfied and full for a long time and, as a result, will reduce cravings drastically. In your transition period as you adjust and reduce the bad foods replacing them with more healthy foods, you might even begin craving healthy foods more.

#5 Eat fiber rich foods

The more you move toward eating whole plant foods, the more fiber you will consume. Fiber helps break food down and also contains a multitude of health benefits. Eating fiber-rich food will make you feel full and satisfied for longer. Since fiber is an essential part of healthy eating, it is discussed in-depth in another chapter.

#6 Ditch processed foods

Processed food almost always contains added sugar or an equally unhealthy sugar substitute. Along with sugar, processed food also contains unhealthy fats, large quantities of sodium, preservatives, and other unhealthy ingredients. It is best to avoid them as much as possible no matter what diet you follow. If you think you might not understand nutrition labels, just think how the food item is made. If it is processed it most likely contains added sugar or simple carbs. If it is a whole plant food, for example a tomato or broccoli, you are good to go.

#7 Avoid fast food

Fast food is addictive because restaurant foods contain a lot of sugar, salt, and fat to give you the desired taste. The enhanced taste does not compare to some home cooked meals. The hungrier you get, the more likely you are to choose a quick fast food run. Going out to eat is always more unhealthy and is typically more expensive than cooking at home. The best tip for avoiding these fast food runs is to meal plan, shop for the meals you've planned so you have enough food at home, and prepare the meals ahead of time. The less often you go out, the more you will get used to natural tastes. As a result, you will begin enjoying natural, home cooked meals more and more.

#8 Don't drink the sugar

One soda contains almost two days worth of the suggested daily sugar intake. So the question here is: Do you really want to drink your calories in sugar? And it is not just sodas! Juices (even 100%) are not a healthy option either because all the fiber is stripped from the juice. So even if it is natural sugar it reacts just like processed table sugar because the juice is a processed food (without fats, fiber, and protein). The better and healthier choice would be eating an apple that contains fructose and fiber. If you can't ditch the soda yet, try the reduction method. Reduce your soda intake each week. You can also try to find more natural replacements. I love to make my own black tea and add lemon Stevia drops. The black tea contains some caffeine and the Stevia will add some natural zero calorie sweetness. They also have different flavors and you don't taste the Stevia much. You don't even have to cook the tea! Simply add the tea bag into cold water and it will diffuse over time.

#9 Start meal planning

While you reorganize your diet, reduce certain foods, and add more healthy options, it is SO important to meal plan. Write down all the meals you want to make for the week: Breakfast, lunch, dinner, and snacks. It might also be helpful to write down a time when you eat these meals and then stick to it. Filling yourself with a well-rounded lunch will help curb cravings in the afternoon. If you don't plan lunch at all you might get really hungry and head toward the quick and easy choice of fast food. Or your hunger may turn into sugar craving and you binge on snacks. Be sure to eat early enough so you don't give cravings a chance. A meal plan will also give you an overview of where you skip the sugar and where you can add your favorite snack without guilt, therefore, you have something to look forward to. Also make sure you only buy the food items on your grocery list. I find it helpful to do grocery pick ups to avoid buying random snacks I see in the store. Plus, grocery pickup helps me spend less money as I don't wander the aisles finding random snacks. Now that your cabinets are full and your meal plan is set, you should be ready to follow a low sugar diet. Remember, if you feel overwhelmed working toward the goal you set out to achieve, you can always take a step back. If you rush the process you might stress yourself and lose motivation!

Troublemaker #2: Oils

Oils are not as healthy as we once believed. Negative health effects are typically based on your current health status, types of oils consumed, and frequency of use. For instance, someone with heart disease should avoid all oils unless otherwise directed by their physician. In one small study[2] patients were put on a whole food plant based diet, meaning no added processed ingredients like oils. Removing processed foods caused the patients' progression of heart disease to be stopped and 70% of the patients saw an opening of their clogged arteries. Oil is not a whole food, it is processed and stripped of macro nutrients (carbs, protein, fiber). Therefore, oil is not as nutrient dense as a whole food. Most oils may be healthier than using ingredients such as butter and some oils are better than others. Olive oil, for example, is better than palm oil or highly processed soybean oil. But coconut oil is just as bad as butter when it comes to saturated fat. The reason why some oils are described as healthy is because of their antioxidant content (vitamin E and K). But you don't need to consume oils to get your antioxidants. There are better whole food options with far more antioxidants, minerals, and fiber, and the alternatives contain less calories.

380 CALORIES
Whole Food vs. Oil

1 cup mashed avocado
vs.
0.2 cup avocado oil

B1 (% RDA)	16%	0
B2 (% RDA)	30%	0
B3 (%RDA)	31%	0
B5 (% RDA)	67%	0
B6 (% RDA)	51%	0
Folate (% RDA)	51%	0
Vitamin A (% RDA)	14%	0
Vitamin C (% RDA)	27%	0
Vitamin E (% RDA)	30%	36%
Vitamin K (% RDA)	54%	44%
Iron (% RDA)	8%	0
Magnesium (% RDA)	22%	0
Potassium (% RDA)	25%	0
Zinc (% RDA)	16%	0
Total fat (g)	35.4	43.6
Protein (g)	4.5	0
Carbs (g)	20	0
Fiber (g)	15.6	0

NUTRIENT DENSITY OF WHOLE PLANT BASED FOOD

1 cup of mashed avocado contains 348 calories compared to 1 cup of avocado oil which contains 1927 calories. And if you try to use the same amount of calories you get 1 cup of mashed avocado for 380 calories and 0.2 cup of avocado oil for the same amount of calories.

The image above shows that you get more nutrients out of 380 calories when consuming whole food compared to oil. Remember, oils are stripped of most nutrients and basically contain only fat.

However, you should still eat healthy fats from whole foods like nuts and seeds. Whole foods like avocados don't contain only fat. They also contains carbs, proteins, minerals, fiber, and vitamins, and they are a balanced food source for healthy fats. Avocados are highest in fat but they contain other macronutrients while oils ONLY contain one macro: fat. Fats are higher in calories. Proteins and carbs contain 4 calories per gram and fats contain 9 calories per gram. Consuming lots of refined oils will also increase the inflammation in your body. Omega 6 fatty acids are healthy on a balanced diet, but they have an inflammatory effect when too much is consumed. Omega 3 fatty acids, on the other hand, have an anti-inflammatory effect. The key is to balance both fats for a healthy diet. An optimal ratio of omega 3:6 is 1:4. This means one part omega 3 per 4 parts omega 6 fatty acids. If you use quality oils here and there that is probably okay. If you are more likely to eat your veggies or salad using olive oil, please do. If you'd like, you can find oil free salad dressing recipes in this book. For frying and cooking you can actually skip the oil. As mentioned before, processed foods contain hidden sugar but also contain low quality oils like canola or soybean. These oils combined with other ingredients in the processed food cause inflammation and should me minimized or cut out completely. You can even find these in vegan junk food. These foods also add unnecessary calories and no nutritional value to your diet. However, I want to point out that I am not suggesting eating zero fat. Fat is essential in a healthy diet, especially for children. I am saying the best sources of healthy fats are whole plant foods.

Here are a few tips to include healthy whole food fat sources in your diet:

1. Add nuts and seeds to your morning oats
2. Add seeds to your smoothies (chia, hemp, flax, etc.)

3. If you snack on carrots or veggies, add nuts to your snack
4. Use salad dressings made with cashews, avocados, or tahini
5. Lunch and Dinner: Make "cheese" sauce with cashews, top Mexican recipes with avocado, or sprinkle hemp seed over your salads and other meals

No Oil Cooking Tips

Tip#1: Oil Free Roasting

You can still make your own potato fries or sweet potato fries. Simply cut them into equally sized strips and spread them over parchment paper or a silicone mat on a baking sheet. Add your seasoning as desired. Set your oven to 400 F and it should take anywhere from 20 to 30 minutes until fully baked. If the food is very dry you can spray on some water, vegetable stock, vinegar, or lemon juice combined with seasoning.

Tip #2: Oil Free Baking

Oils and butters are often used to make pastries moist. Instead, use mashed bananas, apple sauce, or other purees (pumpkin, sweet potatoes).

Tips #3: Oil Free Frying

The best way to get your veggies really crunchy without added oils is using an Air Fryer. This is not a necessary tool since you can just as easily use the oven, but it gets the job done much quicker and makes it more convenient for you. Tofu is one food that is a bit harder to get crispy, so an air fryer is nice. You can make any veggie in the air fryer without oil but you have to experiment with time and heat settings.

Tip #4: Stir-frying, Sauteing, and Browning

For frying, I use about 1/4 cup or less water and heat it up in a stainless steel pan. Then I add the vegetables to fry-steam them on medium heat until they are soft and the water is gone. Once the water has evaporated I add the seasoning and leave them just a bit longer to get some crisp edges. If you water fry onions try adding a pinch of salt. You can also use vegetable stock instead of water. The amount of water depends on the amount and type of food you are making. For example, potatoes take longer so I usually add a lid and steam them until they're almost soft. Then, I remove the lid and let the water evaporate. Lastly, I add the seasoning and let the potatoes brown slightly.

Troublemaker #3: Salt

According to the Centers for Disease Control and Prevention[3], Americans get 71% of their daily sodium from processed food and restaurant food. 9 in 10 US children eat more sodium than recommended and too much can raise blood pressure, risk of heart disease, and stroke. Consuming large amounts of salt causes you to crave strong flavors. As a result, natural unprocessed food tastes bland or boring. According to the Dietary Guidelines for Americans (2015-2020), we should stay under 2300 mg of sodium per day, which is about 0.75 teaspoon of salt per day. Most of us eat much more than this and it is often hidden in processed foods. It's found in many meat products, too. As a rule, if you add 1 teaspoon of salt to a meal that serves 4 and eat one serving of the meal for lunch and dinner, you are fine as long as there is no other salt added during the day. Just like sugar, sodium can be hidden in foods including those that are processed. Hidden sodium can bump up your sodium intake immensely. Change your habits by paying attention to food labels and then start to decrease high sodium foods slowly. If you leave salt out of your recipe and only sprinkle it on top of your food right before eating, you can enhance the salty taste without adding too much salt. Make sure to have a previously measured amount ready if you choose this method. Alternatively, increase the amount of spices withing the recipe to increase flavor.

Troublemaker #4: Pesticides

Pesticides have been linked to certain diseases that cause damage to the nervous system[4] and may cause development delays and hyperactivity, among other ailments. While data is still being collected and is not conclusive, most people find it best to avoid pesticides. Currently, there are over 400 pesticides approved for use in the US. Even though there are limits on how much of each pesticide can be used, there are no limits on how many pesticides per food can be used. The Environmental Working Group tested non-organic produce for pesticides after they had been washed and came up with a list that can be safely consumed (clean fifteen) and other produce that should only be consumed if they are certified organic (dirty dozen). I will say, I don't stress over these findings much. The fear of pesticides should never hold you back from eating fruits and vegetables. The benefits of eating lots of fruits and vegetables are much greater than the risk of possible unsafe pesticide contamination. Be aware, this list changes over time. You can check the newest update on the EWG's homepage[5].

Troublemaker #5: Additives

There are many additives in processed foods that should be avoided. These include nitrates, MSG, artificial sweeteners, and food dyes. The food dye Red 40, Yellow 5, and Yellow 6 have been found to contain carcinogens and red 4 caused cancer in lab animals[6]. Stick to fruits and veggies if you need a boost.

Troublemaker #6: Plastic

Plastic is used to wrap food all the time. Some plastics are better quality than others, but in the end they are not best for health or the environment. The plastics that are used to preserve food can leach harmful compounds into our food and cause detriment to our planet. On average, plastic takes 1,000 years to fully break down. The biggest health threat in the plastic world is BPA which can be found in drink and food packaging for baby products, canned foods, and other wrapped food. BPA is a chemical that disrupts your endocrine system, fertility, and even impacts obesity[7]. In a study of urine samples obtained from 2,517 people, BPA was found in 92.6% of participants[8]. So be sure to look for BPA free items.

To be on the safe side you can switch to all glass containers for storing your food. If you want to stick to plastic make sure to check for the recycling number 1,2,4,5, but avoid the following numbers:

- Recycling number 3: contains PVC or V (Polyvinyl chloride), can be toxic.
- Recycling number 6: contains polystyrene, found to be toxic in animal studies.
- Recycling number 7: contains BPA.

Tips on how to use less plastic:

- If you buy canned food, look for BPA free
- Use your own stainless steel coffee mugs for on the go
- Use BPA free water bottles or get a stainless steel water bottle with BPA free lid
- Store and heat leftovers in Pyrex, ceramic, or glass
- Buy (juice and milk) cartons lined with foil or make your own plant milk and juice
- Get wax paper (bags) to wrap food

Notes

1. American Heart Association. (2018). Added Sugars. Retrieved from https://www.heart.org/en/healthy-living/healthy-eating/eat-smart/sugar/added-sugars
2. Esselstyn, C. B. (2007). Resolving the Coronary Artery Disease Epidemic Through Plant'Based Nutrition. Retrieved from https://onlinelibrary.wiley.com/doi/abs/10.1111/j.1520-037X.2001.00538.x
3. Centers for Disease Control and Prevention. (2019). Salt. Retrieved from https://www.cdc.gov/salt/index.htm
4. Keifer, M. C., & Firestone, J. (2007). Neurotoxicity of pesticides. Retrieved from https://www.ncbi.nlm.nih.gov/pubmed/18032333
5. https://www.ewg.org/
6. Kobylewski, S., & Jacobson, M. F. (2013). Toxicology of food dyes. Retrieved from https://www.tandfonline.com/doi/abs/10.1179/1077352512Z.00000000034?journalCode=yjoh20
7. Vom Saal FS, et al. (2001). The estrogenic endocrine disrupting chemical bisphenol A (BPA) and obesity. Retrieved from https://www.ncbi.nlm.nih.gov/pubmed/22249005
8. National Institute of Environmental Health Sciences. (2019). Bisphenol A (BPA). Retrieved from https://www.niehs.nih.gov/health/topics/agents/sya-bpa/index.cfm

CHAPTER 8: Calories, Calories, Calories

What have you heard about calories? Are your thoughts positive or negative when thinking about calories? Opinions and approaches vary when it comes to the way you manage your diet. Some people count calories for weight loss, others think calories don't matter. It can be tough navigating the intricacies of calories, so let's dive into this fascinating topic.

What are calories and do they differ?

Calories are a unit of energy. Everything we do requires energy. Some activities require small amounts of energy while others require lots of energy. How do we fuel our energy? Food gives our bodies calories and our bodies burn the amount it needs. If there is more energy left, our bodies will store it. Simply put, eating more calories than your body needs for energy makes you gain weight. Even if these calories are all healthy, you'll still gain weight. If you work out the weight gain may be muscle mass.

Here is the difference in calories. Let's take a simple example and compare a doughnut to a plate filled with 1 cup carrots, 1 apple, 10 almonds, and 1 clementine. Both snacks contain 260 calories. The plate contains a much larger volume of food even though it contains the same amount of calories. The doughnut is about 71 g of food and the plate is 423 g of food. Needless to say, the plate will fill you up much more than the doughnut. This is called volume eating.

The other factor we already discussed is nutrient density. 260 calories of whole plant food contains 11 g of fiber, 9 g fat, 5 g protein, B-vitamins, all the vitamin A you need for the day, plenty of vitamin C and E, and also important minerals. The doughnut contains 1 g fiber, 14 g fat (and 6 g of it is saturated fat), 3 g protein, zero vitamins, and zero minerals. Consuming more nutrients per calorie can prevent deficiencies and cravings. Fueling your body with enough quality protein, fiber, and micronutrients will help satiate and satisfy your body for a long period of time.

In summary, eating more calories than your body needs leads to weight gain while eating less calories leads to weight loss. Calories differ in food volume and nutrient density.

Deficient in Calories?

One of the most common vegan mistakes I see is not eating enough calories. Yes, you can be deficient in calories! People who switch from a standard western diet to a whole food plant based diet automatically eat less calories. This is because they eat the same volume as before. Compared to the standard western diet, the same volume of only whole plant foods contain less calories.

Not eating enough calories might make you feel dizzy, tired, and sluggish, and could lead to headaches or mood swings. Not to mention major health risks. Please consider your caloric intake needs while meal planning. All provided recipes and meal plans contain the calorie count. You won't have to count calories for the rest of your life but it is a good idea to get a feel for the right portion size and meal plan that fits your needs.

Determine Your Caloric Intake

Calorie consumption has increased all over the world. In America, the food consumption increased from 2880 calories per day per person in 1961 to 3687 calories per person per day in 2012[1]. In 2013, people were eating 1.5 times as much meat than in 1961, 2.5 times more vegetable oil, and 1.2 times more sugar and sweeteners[2]. Our culture has been increasing food intake, especially foods that are not nutrient dense. Most of us simply don't know how many calories we are eating. Assessing your caloric consumption and determining how many calories you actually need can really help you gain a better understanding of your eating habits.

I like to use the "Body Weight Planner" by the National Institutes of Health[3]. You simply type in your body measurements, activity level, and goals. The program calculates daily caloric intake based on your needs. It includes factors like lifestyle, exercise, age, and weight. This free tool will tell you how many calories you should eat if you want to maintain, lose, or gain weight. Once you know how many calories you need to maintain your weight you can then work on your health goals. For instance, reduce caloric intake to lose weight or increase caloric intake to gain weight. More on that topic in the next chapters.

Another way to determine maintenance calories you need per day is by wearing a fitness tracker with heart rate monitor. This will calculate daily calories burned. You only need to monitor calories burned for a couple of weeks, so it's up to you whether you purchase a tracker or borrow one. If you still aren't sure about this option, try one of these: You can simply start with eating 2000 calories per day for women or 2500 calories per day for men and see if you experience any weight change. If you maintain your weight then you know these are your maintenance calories. The other option would be to track your diet from past daily meals and see how much you have been consuming. If you consumed 2500 calories per day and you gained weight slowly, your maintenance range might be closer to 2300 calories per day. For weight loss you generally want to reduce the calorie intake from your maintenance calories by 200-300 per day and for weight gain you would add 200-300 calories to your maintenance calories. This is a general rule, but there is more to weight loss and muscle gain that we'll talk about next.

Notes

1. ourworldindata.org
2. http://www.fao.org
3. https://www.niddk.nih.gov/bwp

CHAPTER 9: Filled & Fueled Fat Loss

By now you should be able to determine your maintenance calories. As a reminder, these are the calories you need to maintain your weight. If you are unsure, please review the previous chapter about calories.

Typically, you would subtract 200-300 calories (up to 500 calories in some cases) from your maintenance calories to lose weight. The general rule states that you need to burn 3500 calories to lose one pound. Accordingly, you would lose 1 pound per week with a daily caloric deficit of 500. Again, this rule is general and has its limits. There is a point where you can't keep reducing calories in order to lose more weight. If you do not eat enough calories per day for an extended period of time, nutrient deficiencies and weight loss plateaus could result. The better way to create a caloric deficit would be adding an activity or exercise per day. In this chapter we will discuss the risks of a low calorie diet, weight loss plateaus, "cheat" days, and the best exercises for weight loss.

The Risk of Low Calorie Diets

Many people believe if they follow a very low calorie diet they will melt off fat as quickly as possible. I can understand this thought process, but it will not produce the expected results but rather cause the following scenarios:

Risk #1: Weight Loss Plateaus

Restricting calories restricts your body's energy source which puts it into starvation mode. Your body then tries to preserve the energy it still has by slowing down your metabolism. Once your metabolism slows down so does your digestion and nutrient absorption.

If you have made this weight loss mistake, here is how to get out of your weight loss plateau: Calculate maintenance calories and eat accordingly for a week or two. You might think you are gaining weight, but a few pounds extra is not fat gain. This is simply the increased amount of water and food in your system. After this period you can start by cutting 200-300 calories off your meal plan. Another way to beat a weight loss plateau is by adding muscle gain exercises. Increasing muscle mass will give you a strong body and strong bones in the long term and can reduce ailments when you get older. A body with more muscle mass also burns more calories in a resting state even while you are not working out. Strength training during weight loss will also preserve muscle mass while losing fat mass. It is better to lose weight slowly and consistently rather than experiencing constant ups and downs of fast weight loss and plateaus.

Risk #2: Mass Loss Without Fat Loss

The rapid weight loss you often hear about from people following fad diets is mostly the loss of water or fat free mass. After the big drop of weight they still experience fat loss, but the first big drop is not all fat. The end of the fad diet is followed by the typical weight gain, also called the yo-yo effect.

Healthy, gradual fat loss usually happens more consistently than fad diet fat loss and creates long term benefits. A slow process can be frustrating but it is much healthier and more successful. Adding strength training to your routine will help you build muscle mass. Muscles weighs more than fat so you might be losing fat even when you don't see weight loss on the scale. Do not only focus on mass loss.

Risk #3: Nutrient Deficiency

At this time you know whole plant based foods are high in nutrients and volume per calorie. Therefore, these are the best foods for weight loss. Plants will fill and fuel you up without causing you to worry about overdoing the calories. High nutrient intake also helps boost your immune system and reduces inflammation. This anti-inflammatory diet improves nutrient absorption and muscle recovery. Low calorie diets typically lack sufficient nutrients. The risk of nutrient deficiency can increase the longer you are on these diets. You will have a much easier time losing weight with a strong and healthy body. For more tips please refer to the chapter on balancing your meals.

Creating A Weight Loss Diet Plan

In the previous chapters we discussed essential things to know about a healthy balanced plant based diet. Creating a weight loss diet plan is best achieved by focusing on creating a healthy diet first. So the same rules apply: reduce the consumption of processed foods like oils and sugar, balance your meals, focus on whole plant foods, and refer to the food pyramid. The only difference is that your meal plan would create a slight caloric deficit. You eat the same types of food but in smaller portions. Your goal should be to create a diet that can be followed even when you have reached your goal weight. In that case, you can simply increase your food intake without having to change your diet again. This is the lifestyle change approach. In Part 2 of this book I will show you how to transition to a plant based diet. If weight loss is one of your goals, create your meal plan in phase one according to your needs.

Cheat Days

Cheat days are for fad diets. In the transition to a plant based diet you will make small changes over a period of time. This will help you ease into a healthy diet without feeling like you are missing out or restricting yourself. You can create your meal plan with a caloric deficit, include plenty of healthy recipes, leave space for your favorite (vegan) candy bar or restaurant visit, and still be able to lose weight. Your weight loss meal plan will not feel like dieting. Week by week it will get much easier to increase healthy meals and reduce unhealthy meals. Your improved health and lifestyle will be enough motivation for you so you won't feel you need a cheat day.

Best Weight Loss Exercise

There is a difference between aerobic and anaerobic exercise. During aerobic exercise your body uses oxygen to burn carbs and fat for energy (burning calories). During anaerobic exercise your body taps straight into your body's glycogen stores. Both exercise types have their positive effects and both are good for weight loss. Aerobic exercise will also strengthen your cardiovascular system while anaerobic exercise will strengthen bones and build more muscles. Anaerobic exercise is a bit better for fat loss because it also builds muscle mass. Muscles are the only place in your body that burns fat. Increased muscle mass increases your resting metabolic rate (you burn more calories without working out). However, in the end the best workout routine is the one that you stick to. It is generally recommended to exercise 150 minutes per week and you should try different workouts to see which one keeps your motivation. It is also okay to do different types of workouts if you get bored quickly. Aerobic exercises are long endurance exercises that don't get you out of breath quickly like jogging, walking, swimming and cycling. However, if you add some high intensity parts to it you transition into an anaerobic state. Interval training means switching from aerobic training where you breathe easily to high intensity bursts where you breathe heavily. These intervals can be achieved during dancing, jogging, cycling, and other fitness activities. If you have been doing aerobic exercises and you reach a weight loss plateau you should start with adding intervals or other anaerobic exercises like weight training to increase metabolism and fat loss. If you are in the obese and overweight BMI spectrum and have not been doing any exercise at all, you might want to start with walking. Slowly increase the length of your walks then add intense intervals. For example: walk at a normal pace for 5 minutes, then walk fast for 1 minute, normal for 5 minutes, fast for 1.5 minutes, normal for 3, and slow for 1 minute. This would be a good start to interval training for fat burning. You can apply this to other sports and adjust the length and intensity to your fitness level. For overweight people I suggest focusing more on aerobic training first then slowly ease into anaerobic intervals. If you start with long cardio sessions and at the same time reduce your calorie intake significantly, you might get very hungry! Before this gets too hard for you try taking a step back. Do a little less cardio and more strength training or don't cut back too much on your calories.

CHAPTER 10: Plant Powered Muscle Gain

Yes, you do get enough protein on a plant based diet AND you can gain a ton of muscle, as well. Although I am not a professional bodybuilder, I can share some facts if you are considering building muscle on a plant based diet.

Muscle Gain

Most people have a hard time believing that you can build muscle on a vegan diet. They think they need all that animal protein to bulk up. However, Kendrick Farris broke the U.S record in 2016 by lifting a total of 831 pounds in competition. And guess what? He has been on a vegan diet since 2014. So, I would argue it is very possible to gain strength and muscle on a vegan diet. Muscle building is not accomplished by only eating protein. A balanced plant based diet also provides essentials such as antioxidants and anti-inflammatory foods. This helps you quickly recover from your workout so your body is overall healthy. A 2018 review suggests that a greater protein intake of ~1.6 g/kg/day does not increase muscle growth[1]. This means you would not need more than 0.72 grams of protein per pound of weight per day to build muscle. For a man weighing 180 lbs that would be 130 g of protein per day which is easy to get from a balanced vegan diet. However, if you are overweight these numbers do not apply. For an overweight individual, you might want to start with strengthening your muscles while doing interval training to focus more on fat loss while maintaining muscle mass. Once your BMI reaches the normal range of 18.5 to 25 you can increase muscle training.

All whole plant food contains some amount of protein. Here are some high protein foods that are also low in calories:

- 8 oz. seitan: 240 calories, 48 g protein
- 8 oz. firm tofu: 235 calories, 27 g protein
- 4 oz. tempeh: 218 calories, 23 g protein
- 8 oz. edamame: 187 calories, 18.5 g protein
- 1 cup unsweetened soy milk: 70 calories, 7.3 g protein
- 1 cup cooked lentils: 230 calories, 18 g protein
- 1 cup cooked black beans: 241 calories, 17 g protein

Most people are also worried about getting all the essential amino acids with plant based protein. As long as you eat a balanced diet and use different sources, you have nothing to worry about. Quinoa and soy are some of the protein sources that contain a complete amino acid profile.

Here is a quick meal plan example:

Breakfast: 1 cup oats, 1 cup soy milk, 2 T hemp seed, 1 cup berries, and 5 walnut halves (628 calories, 27.3 g protein)

Lunch: Vegan sweet potato chili 1.5 serving (640 calories, 27 g protein)

Snack: ½ cup hummus, 1 medium whole wheat pita bread (360 calories, 14.4 g protein)

Dinner: 1 cup cooked whole wheat pasta, 1 cup cooked lentils, 0.75 cup marinara, 2 cups raw broccoli, steamed (616 calories, 34.4 g protein)

So far we are at 2250 calories and 103 g of plant based protein. If you switch out the lunch above with a seitan BBQ salad (1 cup diced seitan cooked in BBQ sauce and cooled down, served over 1 tomato, 2 cups lettuce, ¼ avocado) you only eat 2000 calories with 128 g plant based protein. I would add a sweet potato smoothie to this meal plan with the BBQ seitan salad to add vitamin A and E which would end up having 138 g of protein and 2320 calories. Another trick is to use lentil pasta or chickpea pasta instead of whole wheat pasta. As you can see, there are many options to create a custom vegan meal plan for gaining muscle. Play around with calories and recipes using an app like "cronometer" for free. For your benefit, I have included another meal plan example with shopping list at the end of this book.

Notes

1. Morton, R. W., Murphy, K. T., McKellar, S. R., Schoenfeld, B. J., Henselmans, M., Helms, E., ... & Phillips, S. M. (2018). A systematic review, meta-analysis and meta-regression of the effect of protein supplementation on resistance training-induced gains in muscle mass and strength in healthy adults. Br J Sports Med, 52(6), 376-384.

PART 2: TRANSITIONING IN 3 PHASES

In Part 1 of this book you've learned the basics of a healthy and balanced vegan diet. Hopefully the information has given you ideas for specific foods you would like to add to your diet. You might be working toward correcting a nutrient deficiency or maybe you have other health goals in mind like weight loss. In Part 2 of this book we will get into the three transition phases. Each phase comes with different challenges and can take anywhere from 1 week to several months.

In Phase 1 we will focus on reducing unwanted foods while adding more whole plant foods to your diet. In Phase 2 we will eliminate most unwanted foods completely. Finally, the last phase is simply troubleshooting issues that might occur and refining your diet further. Please remember, if you feel overwhelmed or you can not stick to your meal plan you can simply take a step back. It is much better to make small changes toward your goal rather than overwhelming yourself and giving up!

You might experience some health improvements right away while others might take months to see. If you are in Phase 2 and you absolutely cannot eliminate all animal derived food, keep it in your diet but reduce frequency or portion size. 90% plant-based eating is better than giving up on the plant based diet altogether. Your accomplishments are up to you and they can also change with time. You can still transition to Phase 3 and refine your diet. If you have given up unhealthy foods and increased your plant intake but you are not 100% plant based you have still made a big, positive change in your life. The more plants you eat, the better!

PHASE 1: Add and Reduce

In Phase 1 you will add more plants to your diet and slowly reduce unwanted foods. This phase will be the most time consuming and challenging. You will learn how to use and manage your time, set your calorie and health goals, and meal plan properly. You will also try new recipes. This phase is all about adding more plant based foods each week and reducing your non-plant food intake without having to eliminate it yet. Transitioning slowly will help you avoid cravings or other side effects like bloating. You will most likely experience improved health and weight. Only take steps that are realistic and able to be transformed into a lasting habit. Here are the steps of phase one:

- Determine foods that should be added or reduced
- Write your goals and meal plan
- Create your shopping list and stock pile list
- Work through the 3 possible challenges for Phase 1
- Prepare easy go-to recipes

Are you ready?

Determining the Foods to Add and Reduce

Below you will find two tables with three columns each. The first table contains all the diet changes that add healthy plant foods to your diet and the second table contains all diet changes that reduce unwanted food. The left column of the table contains the diet change, the middle column contains my notes and suggestions, and the right table offers space to write down the difficulty level. Difficulty level number 1 would mean the diet change is easy to incorporate into your meal plan and number 10 would mean the diet change is too hard. Writing down your difficulty levels is an important step before you move onto meal planning. You can also add your own notes.

ADDING

Diet Change	Notes	Level of difficulty (1=easy, 10= very hard)
Fruits	• Add a serving of fruit to your breakfast • Try to switch your snack with a sweet fruit of choice • Try smoothie recipes	
Vegetables	• Try the dinner recipes from this book • Add a green smoothie • Snack on your choice of vegetable with hummus dip	
Legumes	• Start adding 1 tablespoon of legumes to non-vegan lunch and dinner for one week, then increase • Using the recipes provided in this book, add two plant based dinner recipes to your weekly meal plan • Slowly increase plant based dinner recipes while reducing non-vegan recipes each week	
Healthy Fats	• Make dressings with whole foods like cashews or avocado • Add flax seed and chia seeds to smoothies and oat bowls • Add healthy nuts like walnuts and almonds to oat bowls or have them as a snack. • Eat one Brazil nut per day	
Organize your Plate	To ensure balanced nutrition I suggest filling one half of the plate with vegetables, ¼ with a plant based protein source, and ¼ with a cooked whole grain. Make sure to eat at least 2 cups of cooked vegetables per lunch and dinner and ¾ cup of legumes (or other protein) per lunch and dinner. This is best achieved by following the recipes provided in this book. For breakfast, pick your carbs (oats, buckwheat, bread), your protein, fats (nuts, seeds, soy milk), and plenty of fruits. Try overnight oats or the breakfast smoothie for a balanced breakfast meal. You can also make a hearty breakfast with avocado toast and beans on the side.	

REDUCING

Diet Change	Notes	Level of difficulty (1=easy, 10= very hard)
Reduce meat intake	You can set your own goals: Reduce to 3 times per week, then twice per week, and so on.	
Reduce lunch meat intake	If you consume lunch meat every day, find other lunch alternatives and keep reducing lunch meat intake over time.	
Reduce milk intake	This is as easy as using almond milk instead of cow's milk. You can also find other plant based milk options and see which one tastes best to you.	
Reduce cheese intake	Try new recipes that don't call for cheese and slowly cut back. For sandwiches you can use a hummus spread. There are different flavors to experiment with.	
Reduce other dairy intake (yogurt, hidden dairy like in chocolate)	• Switch to plant based yogurts • Start reading labels to detect hidden dairy	
Reduce egg intake	Eggs are mostly consumed for breakfast so try to make delicious oat bowls every other day. For a hearty breakfast you can try scrambled tofu or a simple avocado toast.	
Reduce unhealthy snacking	Prep better snack options ahead of time (see examples below).	
Reduce fast food	This can be achieved by meal planning and prepping ahead of time.	
Reduce restaurant food	If you enjoy restaurant foods, view my restaurant guide to pick healthier options, but try to reduce it to once per week/month.	
Reduce sugar intake	This is a big one. Read more in the sugar section.	
Reduce soda intake, other sugary drinks like juices	Slowly reduce size and frequency of consumption.	
Reduce oil intake	Refer to no-oil cooking section for practical tips.	
Reduce pre packaged and processed foods	Pay attention to what is a whole food and what is processed. Skip the processed foods more often.	

Healthier snack options can be:

- breakfast smoothie
- simply your favorite fruits and veggies
- apples dipped in peanut butter

- cucumber and baby carrots with hummus
- roasted chickpeas
- chips and guacamole from the stuffed sweet potato recipe
- dried fruits and nuts (watch calories)
- pure chocolate chips
- fruits with vegan chocolate sauce or melted vegan chocolate
- puffed rice cakes with peanut butter (or other nut butter) and fruits
- air fried vegetable chips
- banana rolled with peanut butter into a tortilla and cut into thick slices
- vegan yogurt (watch sugar content) with fruits

Write Out Your Goals and Meal Plan

Formulating your goals before you meal plan helps you stay focused and motivated during the process. It gives your meal plan a clear purpose. The goals can contain weight loss, combating a nutrient deficiency, muscle building, or eating less sugar. The options are endless. You can take all that you have learned in Part 1 of this book into consideration while meal planning. If you have determined your optimal caloric intake, then note it on your meal plan. If you would like to increase a certain micronutrient, add the food rich in said nutrient to your meal plan. Here is an example: For improved iron levels you can plan to eat 1 cup edamame as a snack per day. This would already cover half the iron needed for a women under age 50. You can make this with other veggies and dip as your daily snack.

Another part of the goal setting and meal planning is reviewing your "Adding" and "Reducing" table. Pick the diet change with the lowest difficulty number and add this to your weekly goal. Let's say 4 is your lowest number within the "Adding" table and you placed it beside "trying smoothie recipes." Now find a smoothie recipe from this book and place it in the "snack section" of your meal plan. You can enjoy the same smoothie each day as a snack, try different recipes, or switch between healthy snack options. If you want to try a couple of plant based recipes from this book, add them to your preferred day within your meal plan. Now review your "Reducing" table and see which foods would be easiest to reduce. Let's say you eat eggs twice per week for breakfast but it would be a difficulty level of 2 to reduce your egg consumption to only once per week, then note this in your meal plan. Pick one day where you want to eat eggs and fill the rest of the slots with other plant based breakfast options.

Your meal plan should have some of the slots filled out with new options to try. You can fill the rest of the meal plan with your typical meals. In week two you will build on these changes. Try switching up your breakfast ideas or remove eggs altogether. Maybe something didn't work out well for you in week one. Now is the time to try another approach. Maybe you have tried a couple of dinner recipes from the book. In week two you could add more new dinner recipes. The options are endless and easily adjustable to your needs. The goal is to familiarize yourself with this new lifestyle, implement what works for you, and take small, progressive steps.

The longer you do this the easier it gets, meaning with time you'll see high difficulty levels become less difficult. Below are two example meal plans. Create your meal plan in an order like this.

Meal Plan Example #1:

Goal:	Muscle building
Caloric intake:	2300-2500
Adding this week:	High protein snacks
Reducing this week:	Sugar intake (one snack per day, under 10 g)
Recipes to try:	High protein recipes (XYZ)

Monday Meal Plan Example:
Breakfast: High protein breakfast bowl, 600 cal
Lunch: Sweet potato chili (1.5 servings), 640 cal
Dinner: Creamy tomato pasta (1.5 servings), 700 cal
Snack: PB banana smoothie, 20 baby carrots and 20 pistachios, 420 cal
Total Nutrition: 2400 calories and 100 g protein.

Meal Plan Example #2:

Goal:	Phase 1, slow transition
Caloric intake:	2000
Adding this week:	Smoothies, healthy snacks, healthy breakfast, 1 Tbsp beans
Reducing this week:	Egg intake to once per week
Recipes to try:	Peanut butter smoothie, healthy snack bowl, oat bowl, waffles

	MON	TUE	WED	THU	FR	SAT	SUN
Breakfast	Overnight Oats 500 cal	Overnight Oats	Overnight Oats	Overnight Oats	Overnight Oats	Waffles 500 cal	Eggs and Toast 300 cal
Lunch	Usual lunch + 1 Tbsp beans 500 cal	Usual lunch + 1 Tbsp beans	Usual lunch + 1 Tbsp beans	Fast food	Usual lunch + 1 Tbsp beans 500 cal	Usual lunch + 1 Tbsp beans 500 cal	Usual lunch + 1 Tbsp beans 500 cal
Snack	PB banana smoothie 280 cal	Other Smoothie	Snack Bowl	PB banana smoothie 280 cal	PB banana smoothie 280 cal	Snack Bowl	PB banana smoothie 280 cal
Dinner	Usual dinner 700 cal	Usual dinner 700 cal	Usual dinner 700 cal	Usual dinner 700 cal	Usual dinner 700 cal	Restaurant	Usual dinner 700 cal
Calories	Total calories: 1980						

Tip: To avoid cravings, note the times you get really hungry and try eating just before those times. If you feel like you are starving at 1 pm and this leads to impulse eating, start preparing your lunch at noon. Balance meals with fiber, carbs, fat, and protein to satiate you and help avoid the cravings. Note the times you find it best to eat and incorporate it in your meal plans. If you start a workout routine you might get hungry sooner so pay attention and adjust your eating times accordingly.

Shopping List and Stock Pile List

After creating your meal plan go ahead and write your shopping list. I usually find it easier to write the list on a small piece of recycled paper and have that on hand while going through the grocery store, but use a method that works best for you. Go through each meal and recipe on your meal plan and write down the ingredients. Make sure you write down the exact amount for the serving sizes you need. Then, check your pantry to see if you still have some of the necessary items at home. Now go through your calendar to see if any events or gatherings come up where you need extra food, party snacks, or specific meals.

For the last part of meal planning you will go through a stock pile list that contains everything you need on a regular basis. These items might include dog food, toilet paper, tea, coffee, drinks, milk, or snacks. If there are recipes you repeat each day or week, these ingredients would also be a part of your stock pile list. For example, if you have oats each morning for breakfast, then oats and your typical toppings become a part of the stock pile list. If you don't have a stockpile list yet, you can create one now and change it with time. As your diet changes the stock pile list changes, too. This practice might seem challenging but organization will help you reach your goals much more consistently.

Challenges In Phase 1

Challenge #1: Eating Plant Based With Your Family

If you start a vegan diet for yourself but your partner and kids are not participating, there are a few extra planning steps to consider. Start by including a vegan breakfast and lunch for yourself. Then, with your family, slowly work on switching out the dinner meals. Have a conversation with your family members and see how much they would want to include themselves in the transition. Maybe they are open to reducing meat intake or switching to plant based milk. It is a good idea to consider your family member's eating habits. If they don't mind switching to almond milk, your first successful transition is ditching the cow's milk. While it's not the healthiest choice, your family can try vegan meat substitutes and vegan cheese. They might be more willing to get on board if they have options that suit their tastes. Additionally, add whole food plant based dinner recipes to your weekly meal plan a few times per week starting with one new recipe per week. For the nights they want a meaty dinner there are some meals that are easily adjustable. Let them know that you will eat the vegan meal but you can always add a side of meat or cheese for them. Spaghetti with tomato sauce is vegan and you can easily brown some meat on the side for the rest of the family. You can also blend beans into the marinara sauce for added protein or use meatless crumbles. If you make a Mexican meal, prep all the veggie toppings and cook some chicken for the rest of your family. Your family might follow along with some food swaps, but other swaps you'll only prepare for yourself. If you are not the one cooking, have the person preparing the meal leave the meat out for you and add a plant based protein source on the side. In the beginning phase you might continue eating animal derived food on occasion while including more plants. Although you are not 100% plant based, including more plants in your diet is a very healthy, positive change.

Transitioning kids can be a little more difficult. The smaller they are the easier the transition. Here are some things that helped me bring my toddler along:

I started by making a plate filled with chickpeas, veggies, and fruits as a snack when he was watching TV. This helped him get used to the food without focusing too much on the taste. Whenever he wants cookies, I give these to him at the table and not while watching TV so he is more mindful when eating these snacks. After a while, the healthy snacks have become so normal that he also eats them without watching TV. We also noticed that educating him on the food groups helped him to welcome new healthy foods. We say, "the beans make you really strong, the potatoes really fast, and the broccoli super healthy!" You know your child and know what motivates him. Try different approaches and see what works best for your family. Of course, there are those nights where I try a new recipe and my child will not eat it. By now we understand if he is simply throwing a tantrum or if he really is disgusted by it. I try to take out the food pieces that I know he likes and wash off the spices or sauce. Then serve it with his favorite dip.

Another tip is to include the kids in cooking and baking. While this takes longer and is much more messy it is well worth it. You can explain all the foods that go into the meal and what these foods are good for. When the meal is on the table you can proudly say that the kids made this meal, therefore, they are more likely to eat it. In my opinion, it is also important to explain why we chose not to eat meat and drink milk. I just explain that it is not the best food for us and it is not necessary to eat meat and cheese or drink milk. This reasoning is pretty logical and easily understood by toddlers. I also want to make sure he understands the difference between plant meat and animal meat. Chickenless nuggets and chicken nuggets look the same, therefore, I always tell him the difference. When I prepare chickenless nuggets, I say "chickenless nuggets" or "nuggets." Whenever we attend a birthday party I either bring the plant based version of what is served or adjust his plate with available vegan options. For pizza, I take a napkin and remove the meat and cheese. This process is not as difficult as it seems and has become easy for us these days.

Challenge #2: Your Time, Habits, and Your Motivation

It's important to make time in order to achieve your goals. Although, most people are very busy so they don't add cooking into their schedule. However, long periods of cooking are not necessary for a healthy lifestyle. While you do have to find time to meal plan, shop, cook, and prep, you can do so on little time. Meal planning can take about 20 to 30 minutes per week, shopping can take about one hour per week, and cooking can take 30 minutes per day. Of course, these numbers vary depending on your lifestyle. You can save time or re-organize time to make your plan work. To save time, use grocery pick up services or meal delivery kits, make quick dinner recipes, or subscribe to plant based meal planning services. Then you can also re-organize your schedule to better manage your time. For example, if you know your mornings are too busy, prep your oats the night before. Sometimes small changes in your schedule is all it takes to make healthy eating work.

I can't stress enough the importance of investing in your health. Finding time can be accomplished by reviewing your priorities and activities during the week. Ask yourself why you are so busy? Sometimes it is helpful to write down all the things you do during the day and also note how much time you spend doing these things. Think about which of these things contribute to your goals and align with your purpose. It is okay to cut some things out of your schedule or say no to certain activities. If you don't make time for health now, chances are you have to make time for it later by visiting the doctor or hospital more often. With a healthy body and weight you are not only making your future better, you also get to enjoy the present much more. Whatever your activities are during the day you'll do them with more energy and joy. Experiencing more energy will allow you to accomplish more tasks in a smaller amount of time.

More often today I see people getting sick with diabetes and heart disease in their 30's, 40's, and 50's. Society seems to believe health goes downhill after the age of 30. I started the vegan diet at age 29 and since then my health has drastically improved. My health is much better compared to my 20's. Wouldn't it be awesome to say your health is going uphill in your 30's, 40's, 50's, and beyond?!

I hope reflecting on your time has given you a motivation boost. Now let's talk about changing habits and lifestyle for a moment. In my own life I noticed that understanding the psychology behind my behavior makes it much easier to take control and adjust the behaviors that are causing problems. Changing habits start in the mind. Once we make a decision, we typically act out on this decision. Repeating the same action over and over forms a habit. This habit turns into a lifestyle. In order to change your habits we have to understand that these start with our decision making. Let's look at the root of behavior change. The repetition of a behavior sends signals through pathways to your brain. Imagine a pathway you have made in a forest by walking through the same bushes and grass over and over. Now imagine you stand in front of the forest and you want to take a walk, which way would you go? The pathway would be the easiest. But would it be possible to form another path? Absolutely. Will it take time? Yes. Will it get easier? Of course. Once you have walked the path often enough the grass and bushes are trampled down and walking your new path is easy! Comparing this scenario with eating habits would look like this: A candy bar is super sweet, therefore, the temptation of choosing it as a snack is very high. Since this was an easy decision you start to repeat it over and over. And so you've formed a habit. If you want to replace this habit with a better one, understand that the decision has to be somewhat easy to make. Find a snack that is healthier but that you actually like. Now you have to repeat this habit over and over. You might have to remind yourself along the way to make the same decision. There will be a little resistance at first but after repeating it often enough you make your path more easy to walk and won't have a problem picking the healthy snack. Don't let your emotions fool you. The resistance you feel is only the sign of a previous bad habit, not a sign that you should't make the better choice.

Challenge #3: Budget

The vegan diet can be budget friendly with good planning. But it can also be expensive if you choose mostly processed foods like vegan meat and vegan cheese, or you believe everything has to be non-GMO, organic, or purchased at a specific store. Some exotic ingredients might be harder to get and cost more, as well. But if you stick to seasonal fruits and vegetables, beans, and grains, your meals will not be expensive. In some cases you will pay less for your groceries. Eating beans for protein is much cheaper compared to meat. If you skip the restaurant visits, you will also save money on food. Going to the most frugal grocery store in town keeps my spending between $1.50-$1.90 per plate for a 400-600 calorie dinner. To save even more money go ahead and check the store's ads when you meal plan. See what produce is on sale and plan your meals accordingly. If you find great deals on pantry items, go ahead and stock up. You can also chop and freeze fresh bulk items. Additionally, you can compare prices of nuts and seeds. You might find great deals or be able to order these in bulk online.

4 Easy Go-To Recipes

It is always helpful to have a quick meal option readily available. I like to stock up on marinara, beans, pasta, and frozen veggies. This will make a super easy, yet nutritious meal. Wash and drain the beans then add them with the marinara sauce into a blender and mix until smooth. Warm up the sauce, cook the pasta, and steam some veggies. You can also add riced cauliflower to the paste sauce.

The second recipe is something I plan for busy nights. I simply warm up chickpeas with BBQ sauce then serve it with sliced tomatoes and avocado. Season tomatoes and avocado with salt and pepper and enjoy with the BBQ chickpeas. You can make a similar meal with teriyaki sauce, tofu, rice, and veggies.

For quick Mexican tacos, you can warm up vegan refried beans or other beans with some taco seasoning and top them with lettuce, tomatoes, and guacamole.

I also like to make vegan baked beans with some potatoes and steamed veggies. Most vegetarian baked beans are also vegan. Be sure to read the label. All these recipes are fairly healthy and give you quick options for busy days.

PHASE 2: Eliminate

At the end of Phase 1 you should be eating plenty of fruits, vegetables, legumes, nuts, seeds, and healthy grains. You probably reduced some sugar, oil, and meat consumption. Maybe you made it as far as consuming non vegan food only on rare occasions like parties and gatherings. By now you should feel increased energy levels and also know your optimal portion sizes, eating times, and cooking times. If you feel like you still need to work on any of the mentioned progress, please stay in phase one a while longer. If you are confident, you can progress to phase two.

Foods to Eliminate

In Phase 2, begin eliminating all meat, eggs, and dairy. This phase also comes with a few new challenges that we can tackle one after another. Just like in Phase 1 you will determine which change would be easiest to achieve. For example, some people have a hard time ditching cheese but it is quite easy to swap cow's milk with plant based milk. Therefore, the best change to tackle first would be ditching cow's milk.

Diet Change	Level of difficulty (1=easy, 10= very hard)
Cut out milk	
Cut out yogurt	
Cut out cheese	
Cut out all dairy	
Cut out red meat	
Cut out pork	
Cut out chicken	
Cut out seafood	
Cut out lunch meat (processed meat including hot dogs)	
Cut out eggs	
Cut out snack food that includes animal derived ingredients	

Because you have already increased fiber, adapted your gut bacteria, and reduced animal products, you should not have any side effects from ditching all non plant based foods. If you write down a low number to all the suggestions above you might be able to ditch it all at once. Some people decide to keep one animal derived food (like fish) in their diet for a while longer. Others find it easiest to cut out all at once. You can also cut out one suggestion per week. Again, this really depends on your lifestyle, how much willpower and time you have, and how meal planning works out for you. If you have collected a lot of vegan recipes that you love within Phase 1, the switch to 100% plant based might be very easy at this point.

Challenges In Phase Two

Ditching all animal derived food comes with some new obstacles. For example, you need to start reading labels more carefully, you might experience social challenges, you might wonder what to order in restaurants, and maybe you even experience cravings for meat or cheese. Let's combat these obstacles together!

Challenge #1: Reading Labels

Reading labels to identify healthy and unhealthy foods is an important task. Along with finding added sugar, oil, and salt in a product you also have to watch for added animal-derived ingredients. The easiest way to skip processed foods is to simply stick with the ones that only contain one ingredient. Broccoli only contains broccoli and a pack of oatmeal contains only oatmeal. Different types of cereal on the other hand contain a long list of ingredients. Some packaged and processed foods are still safe to buy so let's discuss certain labels starting with juices. It does not matter if the package of a juice states 100% juice. Juices are a processed food, meaning the fiber and micronutrients are removed. Juices are high in sugar that reacts like refined sugar. The only difference you can make about product quality is buying organic to avoid pesticides. But the sugar content stays the same. Some juices are high in vitamin C but most of the time this is added. It is very easy to get enough vitamin C from a plant based diet. If you struggle with diabetes you should ditch the juices. If you are all around healthy, the occasional juice is fine. Sometimes cheap juices (only 17% juice) contain less sugar than those that are 100% juice. So the ones that you might think are less healthy due to the front label are actually a better choice once you read the full nutrition label on the back. You also have to pay attention to serving size. If one serving size is 8 oz for each product label then you can compare the sugar content. But if one product contains less sugar and the serving size is also smaller it doesn't mean that product contains less sugar. On top of added sugar you also have to watch for added oils. Often, processed foods contain added oils like safflower oil, soybean oil, cottonseed oil, sunflower oil, or corn oil. As mentioned in the chapter about oils (chapter 7), these oils increase inflammation in your body and should be avoided. I also talked about trans fats and hydrogenated oils that should be avoided, as well. Here is an example comparing two types of peanut butter:

LABEL 1

Serv. size	2 Tbsp (32g)
Amount per serving	
Calories 190	
	% DV*
Total Fat 16g	20%
Sat Fat 3g	14%
Trans Fat 0g	
Cholest. 0mg	0%
Sodium 110mg	5%
Total Carb. 7g	2%
Fiber 3g	10%
Total Sugars 2g	
Incl. 0g Added Sugars	0%
Protein 8g	8%
Vit D 0mcg 0% • Calcium 18mg 2%	
Iron 1mg 2% • Potas 201mg 4%	

Ingredients

Peanuts, Contains 1% or Less of Salt.

LABEL 2

Serving size	2 Tbsp. (32g)
Amount per serving	
Calories 180	
	% Daily Value*
Total Fat 15g	19%
Saturated Fat 3g	15%
Trans Fat 0g	
Cholesterol 0mg	0%
Sodium 120mg	5%
Total Carbohydrate 8g	3%
Dietary Fiber 2g	7%
Total Sugars 4g	
Includes 2g Added Sugars	4%
Protein 7g	7%

Ingredients

Roasted Peanuts, Sugar, Contains 2% or less of: Molasses, Fully Hydrogenated Vegetable Oil (Rapeseed, Cottonseed, Soybean), Salt.

When reading labels you have to check two areas: The Nutrition Facts table and the Ingredient list. The two Nutrition Facts labels above show the same serving size (2 Tbsp.). Label 1 contains more fiber and less sugar and sodium. Now let's compare the ingredient list. Label 1 contains peanuts and less than 1% salt. Doesn't look bad at all, does it? Label 2, on the other hand, contains roasted peanuts, sugar, less than 2% molasses (another name for sugar), hydrogenated oils, and salt. Label 1 does not contain added sugar, rather naturally occurring sugar and, therefore, more fiber. Label 2 contains less fiber and added sugar plus more salt and added oils. The Label 1 peanut butter is less processed.

As you can see, there are differences between packaged plant based foods like peanut butters and juices. Now let's get into vegan label reading. Sadly, companies sneak in dairy products in various forms: milk fat, whey, casein, skim milk, and lactose. Some companies use soy lecithin instead of milk lecithin. You find these ingredients in the ingredient list, not in the nutrition label. Some health products that add vitamin D or omega 3 might use them from fish oil, so be sure to check where they are derived. Of course, honey is not vegan so if you avoid it you should check for ingredients like honey, beeswax, royal jelly, and propolis. Other animal derived ingredients are shellac, elastin, keratin, gelatin, collagen, and some food dyes, including #E120 from crushed insects. Obviously, the easiest way to ditch hidden animal food is to stick with whole plant foods. You can always research your favorite snack online to be sure. At the beginning it might seem daunting to read the label of each item. With practice this will get much easier and take less time. Some labels also state "may contain: soy, milk,..." This doesn't mean it's added to the food but the food was manufactured in a facility where these foods are present (potential contamination). This is important to disclose for people with severe food allergies, yet it does not make the food non-vegan.

Challenge #2: Social Situations

In Phase 2 social situations might get more challenging because you'll eliminate all animal derived food from your diet. This means it will be a bit harder to choose what you eat during gatherings, you'll deal with opinionated people, and you'll have to be more organized.

If you are invited to a gathering you can always ask what types of food will be provided. If no vegan options are available you have two choices: Either bring your own food or eat beforehand. If you bring your own food it can be similar to what will be served. If they make hot dogs and sides you can bring vegan hot dogs and sides. Vegan hot dogs are still a processed food and are not healthy but they are a better option than processed meat (carcinogenic) and these gatherings happen only on occasion. If the people at the gathering are not your close friends and you feel uncomfortable asking these details you can eat beforehand. But in my experience you can always find something vegan to fill your plate and be part of the dinner. I once simply had a bun with BBQ sauce. Often there are chips and salsa, veggies, fruit, pasta salad, and more available. If there is pizza I take a napkin and take off the cheese and add veggies on the side but this is not typically considered vegan. It is a good idea to collect some recipes that are easy pot luck meals to make social gatherings a breeze.

When you are at an event and you avoid eating animal derived foods and certain desserts you are sure to get different reactions from the people around you. Good friends are happy for your improved lifestyle while other people might comment, ask, or discuss your new eating habits. Believe me when I say I've heard it all and there are many ways to handle this without creating a stressful situation. First, don't feel offended. Try listening to the other person's point of view first and you might realize they don't truly understand nutrition or they simply believe myths about the vegan diet. You have to determine if the person is really interested in the vegan diet or just wants to argue. Personally, I like to give short and simple answers that sound confident and shut down any potential discussion. It is also a good idea to keep a few answers in mind for common questions and conversations. For example, the question of vegan deficiencies. I had a blood test done and it showed a balanced vegan diet provides all of the necessary nutrition my body needs. So when they ask if I am deficient I am able to say, "No, my blood work is excellent." No explaining necessary. If you have not had a blood test done yet you can simply say you are trying to eat more plants to see how it would affect your health. Be transparent about your motivations and most people will not dig or instigate as much. Another conversation piece is the protein question. I tell people I get 70-100 g plant based protein a day from plants without any shakes or supplements. Done. I also like to mention Kendrick Farris who broke the U.S record in 2016 by lifting a total of 831 pounds after committing to a vegan diet in 2014. Sometimes I'm asked why I changed my diet. Simple, for my health and for environmental reasons. General, yet to the point. I think it is good to give answers that show it was my personal decision to improve my life. This makes it less offensive and the other person will not feel like you are suggesting they change their diet, too. Therefore, I usually don't give a speech about the benefits of a plant based diet and I keep my answers more personal. Don't try selling veganism because it can quickly become a religion. Food religions are not good for anyone. Another response vegans often hear is, "I could never do this because..." Most people believe they are "just meat eaters" and so it has become a part of their identity. Telling them how bad meat is will not change the way they think. My answer to this is simply, "Ah, okay." If I feel like someone is really desperate to make a diet change, I encourage them to eat more fruits and veggies, ditch processed foods, and reduce meat intake. This is great health advice for any diet type and would still bring individuals closer to a whole food plant based diet without trying to push them to be vegan. Don't feel the need to convince anyone. Know that you are doing this for your personal health. No one is going to take care of your health care bills so it does not matter what they think or say. Also keep in mind, social relationships should not suffer because of different eating habits.

Challenge #3: Restaurants

Vegan or not, restaurant food is filled with salt, sugar, and fat. Eating at restaurants will often train your taste to only want these types of foods. As a result, homemade steamed veggies taste boring and you might find yourself craving restaurant foods even more. Eating out less often will help curb cravings with time and can be a part of the habit changes you created in Phase 1. In Phase 2 you are ditching all animal products. Now your restaurant choices may be limited and at some restaurants you will have to change your meal orders. Most restaurants have vegetarian options but not all have vegan options. Fear not, there are still many options available to you. When my family first started a vegan diet we rarely went out to eat. We didn't know what to order and we weren't sure what ingredients were in the food we wanted to eat so we chose to avoid the hassle. While this saved lots of money and was much healthier, we still wanted to enjoy the luxury of eating out. Often for the vegetarian option, it's as easy as telling the waiter "no cheese." For example, you can order vegetarian fajitas and ditch the cheese and sour cream. You ALWAYS have to say this because restaurants automatically add cheese to these meals. If your partner orders the same meal simply repeat the whole order and say, "NO CHEESE" again, just to be clear. Trust me, many restaurants will get it wrong. Be sure to double check the meal ingredients for butter, eggs, milk, or any other non-vegan additions. Ordering vegan in restaurants will often save you on calories, as well. If you order a chicken parmesan meal at an Italian restaurant, your dinner contains over 1,000 calories. If you choose the whole wheat linguine, marinara, and steamed veggies (broccoli) you are at 575 calories, 21 g of fiber, and 24 g of protein. This makes a huge difference in your nutrition. Mexican restaurants are my favorite choice to eat vegan. They have beans for protein and usually offer steamed veggies, salsa, rice, corn, and guacamole. What could be better? If you go to sandwich places, simply fill your sandwich with lots of veggies as if you're preparing a salad in a bun. Top this with a vinaigrette or mustard. Pizzas are also easy to customize. Many original pizza dough recipes are vegan but it is better if you check the ingredient list first. Then top with your favorite veggies and skip the cheese. Some garlic dips are vegan, too, so spice up your pizza with it. A go-to meal at Asian restaurants is steamed veggies, rice, and edamame (high in protein). You can also try veggie sushi without the sauce on top. These days, most burger restaurants carry a veggie burger or meat replacement option. Just make sure they don't add cheese, mayonnaise, or a burger sauce that is non-vegan. Sometimes they put the vegan burger option under "sandwiches." You can also create a meal choosing multiple sides or by choosing foods they provide within other meals. The good news is that the plant based movement is becoming more popular so more vegan options are available in a growing number of restaurants.

Challenge #4: Cravings

There are two main ways to avoid cravings: Plan and prepare your meals and choose balanced, nourishing meals. If you eat junk food and your body does not get proper nutrition it will crave even more food. If you choose a low carb or low calorie diet, your body will crave food. If you wait too long to eat your cravings will increase. To avoid general cravings make sure to meal plan properly, balance out your meals, and eat before you get really hungry.

You might also experience specific meat or cheese cravings in the beginning stages of your vegan journey. Know that this is normal because your prior lifestyle included these things for a long time. It's what you were adjusted to eating so your body will initially trigger these cravings. When I craved meat or cheese I reminded myself why I chose this lifestyle and it helped me overcome those cravings. I choose to remember all the health and environmental benefits. I also acknowledge that the cravings come from a habit I formed in the past and they are not a sign that I am made to eat meat. To say it plainly: I do not miss out on or give up anything. I focus on the food I get to eat, not on the food I am not eating.

There are many plant based meat alternatives for burgers, nuggets, strips, and anything else your heart desires that can be used to curb your cravings. Find your favorite plant based meat alternative and have it available in your freezer during your transition phase. With time, you will find more and more tasty whole food plant based recipes that hit the spot while reducing your desire for processed vegan food. I can assure you that the cravings will subside. Change and growth occur when you face challenges and power through adversity.

PHASE 3: Refine and Troubleshoot

At the end of Phase 2 you should be comfortable and consistent with your plant based diet. You have overcome most obstacles. You have confidence at social gatherings. You've also created a collection of favorite recipes and know what works and doesn't work for you. Personally, I realized we do not like quinoa so I won't try new recipes including quinoa anymore. Rice works better for us so this is what we will stick to. There is no point trying to force certain health foods into your life. Phase 3 is not a transitional phase that ends, but rather a lasting phase of continuous improvements and troubleshooting.

Refine and Adjust

While your eating habits should not look like a roller coaster of healthy and unhealthy eating, it is quite normal to have smaller fluctuations. Outside factors might cause us to adjust our lifestyle and inside factors might cause us to refine our lifestyle. Christmas time can lead you to eat more food, life gets busy and your meal prep schedule gets off track, or other lifestyle changes happen. Life events can throw off our flow of meal planning, cooking, and other healthy habits. That's when you take time to reflect and adjust.

Maybe an internal factor or goals have changed and you want to refine your lifestyle with these things in mind. You can refine your lifestyle towards increasing a certain nutrient, include a certain plant food more often, or increase calories for a more active lifestyle. The options of refining are endless. However, this is not without risk. Some people keep refining their diet to such an extreme that it becomes an eating disorder. Because the vegan diet is considered "extreme" when compared to the standard western diet, the concern of eating disorders such as "Orthorexia" arises. Orthorexia, not officially recognized yet, is an obsessive concern about the relationship between food and your health. Veganism can hide a very restrictive diet, meaning people with Orthorexia tend to choose a restrictive vegan diet or vegans fall into the obsessive behavior when trying to eat a healthy diet. If you choose the vegan diet but add more restrictive rules to it, the diet can become unhealthy pretty quickly. It gets dangerous if you are trying to eat as clean as possible at all times. Reflect on your purpose and recognize if your healthy eating 'rules' bring out fear or if they keep you away from social events. Other signs of obsessive behavior include: reoccurring cycles of detox, frequent fasting, and continuously adding more rules to your diet. A vegan diet is restrictive when compared to the standard western diet, but naturally and nutritiously the vegan diet is not restrictive. Think about it, the vegan diet cuts out all animal derived foods but it does not cut out essential food groups like fats or carbs.

In the beginning phases of a vegan diet you learned a lot about the diet, you have tried new recipes, and you may have become passionate about all the health benefits you are experiencing. That's normal. Within your journey you might cut back on certain foods that cause sensitivities, allergies, or discomfort. That's normal, too. You might have found your energy levels are more consistent if you cut out sugar completely or you read about a superfood and started including it in your diet. Maybe you realize that you get heartburn from a certain food and reduce consumption of that food. Mindful eating, eating with purpose, and creating meaningful dietary guidelines can make it much easier to stick to a long term healthy diet. These guidelines provide security and clarity when meal planning or going out to eat. Use caution, there is a difference between discipline and obsession.

Here are some signs your relationship with food may be unhealthy:

1. You are reaching for multiple supplements and or other remedies
2. Your thoughts revolve around food and health most of the time (unless it is your job)
3. You feel superior because of your eating style
4. You feel the need to "convert" others to your eating habit
5. You fear going to social events because of the food choices
6. You believe there is only one way to eat right or healthy
7. You stop feeling hungry or lose connection with your body
8. You are very hard on yourself if you eat outside of your 'rules'

Troubleshoot Your Diet

If you have been on the vegan diet for a while but still struggle in certain areas, or start struggling, now is the time to troubleshoot. Some people start a vegan diet and feel great. Others experience some side effects or long term deficiencies. Don't give up on a plant based diet. Here are some of the most common side effects to look out for:

Food sensitivities

Sometimes sensitivities are triggered by higher quantities of certain foods. If you think you show signs of a food intolerance you can get tested by your health provider, create a food diary and perform a self analysis, or try an elimination diet. An elimination diet is simply removing all suspected allergens from your diet to see if the symptoms go away. Then start introducing one of the eliminated foods back into the diet for 3-6 days and see if you stay clear of any symptoms. If you do, you can introduce the next one. This way you can find out which food triggers the intolerance and you can find a substitute.

Bloating

Bloating is typically caused by quickly introducing a large amount of fiber into your diet. Please refer to the fiber section in this book for details. If you follow all the tips for bloating and still experience discomfort, you might be reacting with a food sensitivity.

Sluggishness, experiencing low energy, and headaches

The most common causes of sluggishness, low energy, and headaches are:

- a calorie deficiency
- unbalanced meals
- lack of macro and micro nutrients

As already explained, plant based food has a higher volume for less calories. It's easy to think we eat a lot when, realistically, we are not eating enough. Not eating enough food will make you feel sluggish. Most deficiencies come from not including all macro nutrients into your diet. Don't go low fat or low carb. Another common mistake is not including a plant based protein source with each meal. These subjects are thoroughly discussed in Part 1 of this book and I highly recommend going though it again if you experience any of these side effects. Another great tool is a nutrition tracking app like cronometer. With this tool you can add everything you eat during the day and see what macro or micro nutrient you are low in. If you experience sharp acute side effects or chronic side effects please speak to your healthcare provider.

PART 3: RECIPES

Each recipe was created with the food pyramid in mind. All dinner and lunch recipes contain a plant based protein source. You can adjust each recipe to your needs. For example, you can add more veggies, more protein, or more calories. Before I get into the recipes, I would like to talk about certain foods and their purpose while also explaining a few recipe options.

Under each recipe you can find extra notes or tips. I use "t" for teaspoon and "T" for tablespoon. You can use the ingredient list and cut everything in half to serve 2 or double everything for a larger portion size or more portions. Most of the recipes are freezer friendly. You can also use parts of one recipe and add it to another recipe. For example, use the salsa and guacamole recipe from the stuffed sweet potato recipe for tacos.

Cheese

You can make your own parmesan cheese by grinding cashews with nutritional yeast. Top any recipe with this mix. You can also buy vegan cheese for an added topping. I did not include vegan cheese as an option because it is a processed food. But if adding ingredients to your food becomes more desirable, go ahead and sprinkle some vegan cheese on it. Try different brands because some vegan cheese brands do not melt easily.

Salt

If you are trying to ditch salt for health reasons you can leave it out of the recipes and increase the amount of other spices.

Pizza

This book does not include a pizza recipe, but you can buy your favorite pizza dough and top with pizza sauce, veggies, and vegan cheese. The pizza dough that comes in rolls in the freezer section is the best I've tried so far. I did not like the dough from the bread section. Make sure to read ingredient labels. Some ready made pizza dough products are not vegan.

Tofu

There is normal, firm, and extra firm tofu. If you use tofu to make a cream sauce, use normal tofu. If you use tofu to eat as chunks, use extra firm tofu. You can use the oven or an air fryer to make tofu crisp.

Vegetable Stock

I always buy vegetable stock powder as an additional seasoning. You can use this for any recipe to enhance the taste. You can also omit and increase the other spices. Some vegetable stock powders contain unhealthy fillers and too much sodium, so be aware of this when buying.

Kitchen Tools

For soups I use a hand blender, for sauces and smoothies I use either a smoothie maker or a food processor. Before you buy your kitchen tools do some research and also make sure it is big enough for the job. I had a small food processor and had to make sauces in 3 batches. The bigger blender will save you a significant amount of time. A larger all-in-one machine might be your best option.

Oil Free (OF)

Most recipes in this book are oil free.

Gluten Free (GF)

There are a lot of gluten free options throughout the recipes. However, you can change any recipe in this book to make it gluten free. The overnight oats and smoothies are all gluten free and for any pasta meal you can buy gluten free pasta like lentil pasta, chickpea pasta, or rice pasta. I like to use Asian rice noodles instead of spaghetti to make the spaghetti or linguine dish gluten free. For the sandwiches you can get gluten free bread or find other options.

Calories

If one serving of a lunch or dinner recipe contains 300 calories, the meal will most likely not satiate you unless it is supposed to be a side or a small lunch. Therefore, I suggest increasing the serving size so you are full after the meal. You can use this same tip to find other new recipes as well. It is best to eat at least 400 calories, better 500 or 600 calories for lunch and dinner. This will provide enough calories to maintain energy, nutrients to avoid deficiencies, and volume to curb cravings.

Serving Sizes

Each recipe shows how many people it serves. If a recipe serves 4 then you would have to split it into 4 equal parts to get the nutritional value noted for each recipe. Typically, one serving size measures 2-3 cups of food. Recipe nutrition values are more exact by splitting them up into equal parts.

One Pot

Most of the one pot recipes can be made in a pressure cooker. I usually set the setting to stew – high – 5 minutes and close the valve for all recipes. This makes dinner super easy! You can also make them in a slow cooker.

Allergies

If you have a peanut allergy, you can substitute peanut butter with tahini. Substitute soy milk with cashew milk which is a little creamier than almond milk. Some cream sauces are made with tofu but you can leave out the tofu and make it with cashews.

Smoothies

You can switch out the fruits, nuts, seeds, and plant milk within your smoothie and experiment with your own recipes. Generally, you have to add more sweet or citrus fruits than the beans or vegetables. That way you won't taste them. Please drink your smoothies slowly to give your body time to absorb all the nutrients and the fruit sugar.

BREAKFAST AND SMOOTHIES

Carrot Cake Oat Bowl

Serves 1 | 10 Minutes | GF | OF

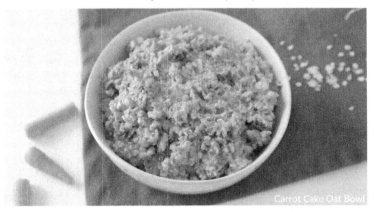

INGREDIENTS:

- 3/4 cup whole oats
- 1/2 cup shredded carrots (6 baby carrots)
- 1 T chia seeds
- 2 T chopped walnuts
- 1/2 t cinnamon
- 1 cup soy milk
- 2 t maple syrup (optional, omit if you want less sweetness/no added sugar)
- 1/4 t vanilla extract
- 2 dashes nutmeg
- 1/4 cup raisins
- 1 Brazil nut

INSTRUCTIONS:

Combine and stir all ingredients in a container and let sit in the fridge overnight. You might have to add more liquid next morning if the mix seems too dry. Alternatively, add all ingredients into a small pot and heat for 3-5 minutes. Stir occasionally.

Per Serving: 560 Cal | 82 g Carbs | 16 g Fiber | 20 g Protein | 19 g Fat

Easy Balanced Oat Bowl

Serves 1 | 10 Minutes | GF | OF

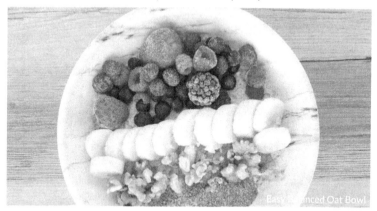

INGREDIENTS:

- 1 cup quick oats
- 1 cup almond milk
- 1/2 cup mixed berries
- 1 banana
- 1 Brazil nut
- 2 T chopped walnuts
- 1 T milled flax seed

INSTRUCTIONS:

Combine everything in a bowl and enjoy. You can prep this the night before for a quick and easy breakfast.

This oat bowl provides great nutrition: 5.8 mg iron, 3.9 mg zinc, 963 mg potassium, 200 mg magnesium, and more.

Per Serving: 620 Cal | 96 g Carbs | 16 g Fiber | 18 g Protein | 21.4 g Fat

Peanut Butter Chocolate Oats

Serves 1 | 5 Minutes Prep Time | GF | OF

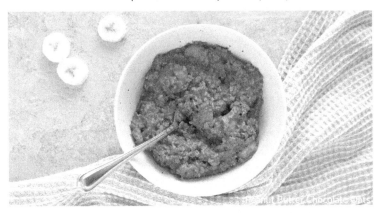

INGREDIENTS:

- 1 cup oats
- 1 cup almond milk
- 1 T peanut butter
- 1 T ground flax seeds
- 1 banana
- 1 Brazil nut
- 2 T cocoa powder
- maple syrup (optional)

INSTRUCTIONS:

Combine everything in a bowl and mix thoroughly. You can heat this mix up for 2-3 minutes and it will thicken. You can also prep this the night before and leave in the fridge overnight. Then add more milk in the morning if the oats are too thick. Note that this is not sweetened. If you like you can add some maple syrup.

Per Serving: 630 Cal | 95 g Carbs | 18 Fiber | 21 g Protein | 24 g Fat

No Bake Energy Bites

10 Balls | 15 Minutes | GF | OF

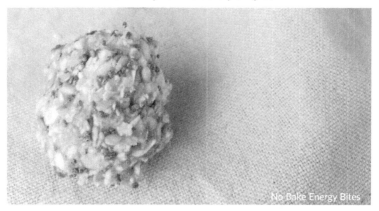

INGREDIENTS:

- 1/2 cup oats
- 1/2 cup nuts (almond, walnut, cashews,...)
- 1/2 cup chopped dates (or other dry fruit)
- 2 T chia seed
- 2 T flaxseed
- 3 T maple syrup
- 1-2 T peanut butter

INSTRUCTIONS:

Add everything except the syrup and the peanut butter to a food processor and chop. Then add the rest of the ingredients and 'massage' it into the mix until everything is sticky enough to form the balls. If you have a hard time forming the balls simply add more syrup or peanut butter. This recipe makes 10 balls.

One Ball: 136 Cal | 18 g Carbs | 3.2 Fiber | 3.7 g Protein | 6.4 g Fat

Easy Oat Waffles

1 Waffle | 10 Minutes | GF | OF

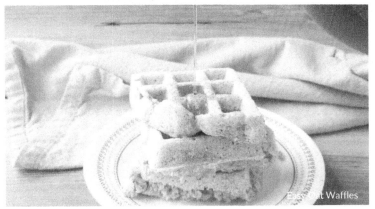

INGREDIENTS:

- 1 cup oat flour (or ground oats)
- 3/4 cup almond milk
- 1/4 t baking powder
- dash of salt
- 1 t ground flax seed
- Waffle Maker

INSTRUCTIONS:

Mix all ingredients together and add to the waffle maker. Make sure the waffle maker is heated up all the way and the green light is on (green light goes off once you add the mix). Then bake until the green light comes on again.

You can use medium or high heat depending on the desired browning. The cooking time depends on your settings. Make sure to use a quality non stick waffle maker and only open it when the light turns green again. The recipe above makes one large Belgian waffle. Depending on the size of your waffle maker you might get different serving sizes. You can always double up the ingredients to make more waffles. I also had good results using ground oats, flax seed, and almond milk only. You can top this with jelly, chocolate chips, syrup, and more.

One Serving: 495 Cal | 83 g Carbs | 12.8 Fiber | 17.3 g Protein | 10.8 g Fat

Tropical Sunrise Chia Pudding

Serves 1 | 5 Minutes Prep Time | GF | OF

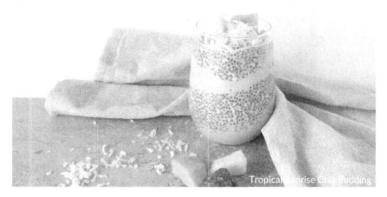

INGREDIENTS:

- 3 T chia seeds
- 3/4 cup almond milk + 2 T coconut flakes (or use 3/4 cup coconut milk)
- 1 cup frozen tropical fruit mix (or use your favorite tropical fruits)
- Optional: 1 cup soy milk

INSTRUCTIONS:

Add the chia seeds, almond milk, and coconut flakes (or just use coconut milk) in a jar, stir, and let sit overnight. To make the layers, use one cup of frozen tropical fruit blend and puree it in a blender with 1 cup of soy milk. It becomes a slushy-like texture if you use frozen fruits and this should be eaten right away.

To make the puree with fresh (not frozen fruits) start out by using less milk. Now layer the puree with the chia pudding. If you want to make this chia pudding for meal prep I suggest just topping the chia pudding with the fruits and store in the fridge. The nutritional value refers to the recipe using almond milk + coconut flakes and soy milk for the puree. You can sweeten this with vanilla extract or maple syrup if desired.

Per Serving: 400 Cal | 41 g Carbs | 18 Fiber | 14.5 g Protein | 21 g Fat

Black Forest Cake Smoothie

Serves 1 | 10 Minutes | GF | OF

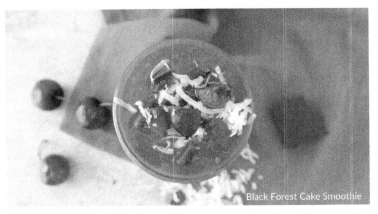

INGREDIENTS:

- 1 T chia seeds
- 1 banana
- 1/2 cup almond milk
- 10 pitted cherries
- 2 T cocoa powder (unsweetened)
- 1 hand full (or 1 cup) fresh baby spinach

INSTRUCTIONS:

Add everything into a high quality blender and mix until smooth.

Per Serving: 250 Cal | 52 g Carbs | 13 g Fiber | 7.5 g Protein | 6.5 g Fat

Easy Berry Breakfast Smoothie

Serves 1 | 5 Minutes Prep Time | GF | OF

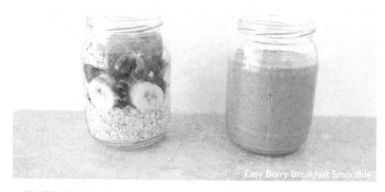

INGREDIENTS:

- 1/2 cup oats
- 1.5 cups almond milk
- 1 T chopped walnuts
- 1 T milled flax seed
- 1 cup berries (frozen or fresh)
- 1 banana
- 1 Brazil nut
- optional: spinach

INSTRUCTIONS:

Add everything into a blender and mix until smooth. You can easily prep this smoothie mix the night before and store in a glass jar (I use recycled sauerkraut jars). The next morning dump the mix into your blender and add the almond milk. You can also use soy milk for added protein. You can add more oats if you like but start with 1/2 cup first to see how it tastes. If you add more it might taste too powdery.

Per Serving: 480 Cal | 76 g Carbs | 12 Fiber | 12 g Protein | 16 g Fat

High Protein Green Smoothie

1 Serving | 5 Minutes | GF | OF

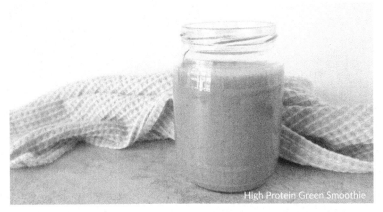

INGREDIENTS:

- 1 banana
- 1 cup spinach (fresh baby)
- 2 T hemp seeds
- 1.25 cup soy milk (unsweetened, original)
- 1/2 cup black beans (rinsed)
- 1 dried date (stone removed)

INSTRUCTIONS:

Simply add all ingredients into a blender and mix until smooth. You can also leave out the date if you don't want to sweeten the smoothie. You can get whole dates or dried date junks.

One Serving: 450 Cal | 65 g Carbs | 22 Fiber | 24 g Protein | 13 g Fat

Immunity Boosting Smoothie

1 Smoothie | 10 Minutes | GF | OF

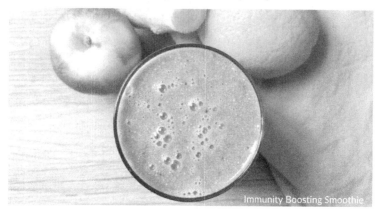

INGREDIENTS:

- 1 apple, without the core
- 1 orange, peeled
- 1 cup or handful baby spinach
- 10 raw, unsalted cashews
- 1/4 t cinnamon
- 4 dashes turmeric
- 1 dash black pepper
- 1 cup water (or plant milk)
- small piece of ginger (a half inch slice)

INSTRUCTIONS:

Simply put all ingredients into a blender and mix. If your blender is not powerful enough, grind the ginger beforehand instead of adding a whole piece.

The cashews are high in zinc. Turmeric and cinnamon have anti-inflammatory properties. The apple is high in flavenoids. The orange is high in vitamin C. Ginger and spinach are packed with nutrients and anti oxidants.

One Serving: 250 Cal | 47 g Carbs | 9.1 Fiber | 5.6 g Protein | 7.7 g Fat

Grapefruit Banana Green Smoothie

1 Smoothie | 8 Minutes | GF | OF

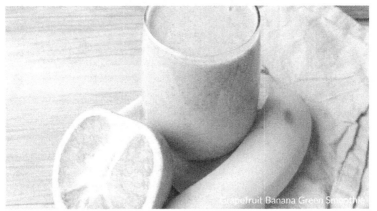

INGREDIENTS:

- 1 grapefruit, peeled
- 1 banana
- 1 cup almond milk unsweetened (or vanilla)
- 1 T chia seeds
- 1 T chopped walnuts
- 1-2 cups spinach
- optional: cinnamon, turmeric

INSTRUCTIONS:

Add all ingredients into a blender and mix until smooth. You can add more spices or nuts and seeds as desired.

One Serving: 355 Cal | 62 g Carbs | 9.1 Fiber | 8.7 g Protein | 11.4 g Fat

Sweet Potato Green Smoothie

1 Smoothie | 8 Minutes | GF | OF

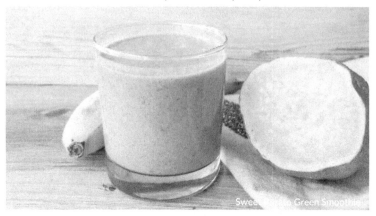

INGREDIENTS:

- 1 Banana
- 1/4 cup sweet potato cubes
- 1.5 cups spinach
- 1 cup almond milk (unsweetened)
- 1 T peanut butter (unsweetened)
- 1 T chia seeds

INSTRUCTIONS:

Add everything into a blender and mix until smooth. Drink your smoothie slowly.

One Serving: 350 Cal | 51 g Carbs | 10.3 Fiber | 10 g Protein | 14.6 g Fat

SALADS AND SANDWICHES

Caprese Pasta Salad

Serves 4 | 20 Minutes | OF

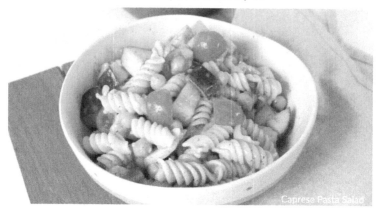

INGREDIENTS:

- 8 oz. dry whole wheat penne pasta or fusilli
- 1 can chickpeas, rinsed but save the drained liquid for dressing
- 1 cucumber, cubed
- 1 pint (40) cherry tomatoes
- 1 avocado
- dashes of pepper
- 1/2 t salt
- 2 t balsamic vinegar
- 1/2 t basil, dried
- 1/2 t oregano, dried

INSTRUCTIONS:

Cook pasta according to the package instruction then rinse with cold water until cool. In the meantime cut the cherry tomatoes in half, cube the cucumber and 1/2 of the avocado. For the dressing use the other half of the avocado, the liquid from the canned chickpeas, salt, pepper, balsamic vinegar, and herbs and mix in a blender until smooth. Add all ingredients in a large bowl and mix in the dressing. Each serving should be around 2.5 cups. You can use gluten free pasta to make this meal gluten free.

Per Serving: 380 Cal | 66 g Carbs | 13 g Fiber | 14 g Protein | 8.7 g Fat

Roasted Vegetable Salad (Autumn Edition)

Serves 1 | 25 Minutes | GF | OF

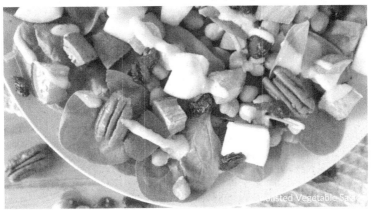

INGREDIENTS:

- 2 cups fresh baby spinach
- 1/2 medium sweet potato, cubed
- 0.75 cup (1/2 can) chickpeas, drained and rinsed
- 1 t thyme
- salt to taste
- 1 T dried unsweetened cranberries
- 5 pecan halves
- 1/2 apple, cubed
- Dressing: Choose from the following dressings. The Italian dressing and the mustard-maple dressing work well.

INSTRUCTIONS:

Spread the rinsed chickpeas and cubed sweet potatoes on a baking sheet and sprinkle with salt and dried thyme. Then bake on 425 F for 15 minutes (until sweet potatoes are soft). In the meantime, assemble the salad and prepare the dressing. You can let the chickpeas and sweet potatoes cool if you like. Then add to your salad and drizzle with the dressing. This recipe makes one salad. You can make more servings to prep for the week. Change ingredients and adjust this salad to your needs and taste. The nutritional values are for one salad with the Italian dressing.

Per Serving: 400 Cal | 71 g Carbs | 16 g Fiber | 14.6 g Protein | 9 g Fat

3 Salad Dressings

5 Minutes | GF | OF
You can adjust the spices and herbs to your taste!

CAESAR DRESSING

- 3/4 cup unsalted raw cashews (soaked in warm water for 15 minutes)
- 3/4 cup water
- 1.5 t apple cider vinegar
- 1.5 t Dijon mustard
- 1.5 t garlic powder
- 1-1.5 t salt
- 5 dashes of pepper
- 1.5 t maple syrup

Cover the cashews with warm water and soak for 10 to 15 minutes. In the meantime, prepare all your veggies. You can use this Caesar dressing on any salad and vegetable. Then drain the cashews and add all ingredients into a mixer and blend well (including the 3/4 cup of water). Drizzle the dressing over your salad and enjoy!

EASY ITALIAN

- 4 oz tofu (firm)
- 1/4 cup water
- 2.5 tsp. red wine vinegar (or apple cider vinegar)
- 0.5 cloves fresh garlic
- 1.5 tsp. dried herbs de Provence (Italian seasoning)
- optional: salt and pepper to taste

Add all ingredients in a blender and mix until smooth. You can always adjust the spices or add salt if desired. If you store this dressing in the fridge, it might separate. Please shake before use.

MAPLE MUSTARD

- 4 oz. firm tofu
- 1/4 cup water
- 1/2 t salt
- 2 t red wine vinegar
- 2 t Dijon mustard (or normal mustard)
- 1 t maple syrup

Add all ingredients to a blender and mix. This recipe serves 4. Each serving is about 4 tablespoons and covers a large salad that equals 4-5 cups. Store leftovers in the fridge and shake before use. You can adjust the ingredients to your taste.

Easy Lentil Salad

Serves 4 | 15 Minutes | GF | OF

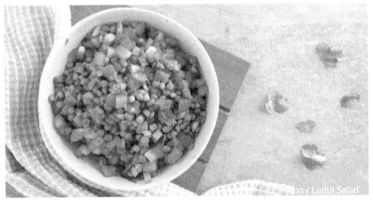

INGREDIENTS:

- 2 cans (3 cups) cooked canned red lentils (drained)
- 2 red bell peppers, finely cubed
- 1/2 bundle cilantro, chopped (or fresh parsley)
- juice of 1/2 lemon
- 1 clove garlic
- 1/4 medium onion, finely cubed
- 1/4 t salt pepper to taste
- 1/2 - 1 t thyme (optional)

INSTRUCTIONS:

Drain the lentils (you don't have to rinse) and combine with the other ingredients. Add more spices as desired.

You can use this for lunch and increase serving size as needed. You can bring this recipe to parties or enjoy with some oven roasted potatoes.

Per Serving: 202 Cal | 38 g Carbs | 6.3 g Fiber | 12 g Protein | 0.2 g Fat

Homemade Hummus

10 Minutes | GF | OF

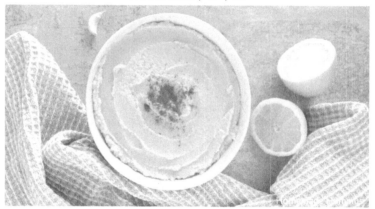

INGREDIENTS:

- 2 cans chickpeas, drained and rinsed
- juice of 1 lemon
- 1 clove garlic
- 1 t peanut butter or tahini
- 1/2 t cumin
- 1/4 t salt (optional)
- 1 cup water
- paprika powder to sprinkle (optional)

INSTRUCTIONS:

Blend all ingredients using 1/2 cup of the water first. You can add more water slowly if it doesn't blend. You can also adjust the spices to your desire. I use peanut butter (oil free, no sugar added) instead of tahini and it tastes great. You can also reduce the amount of peanut butter if you like but it makes the hummus more creamy (instead of using oil).

One Batch: 854 Cal | 140 g Carbs | 38 g Fiber | 45 g Protein | 15.6 g Fat

The hummus can be stored in the fridge for at least one week.

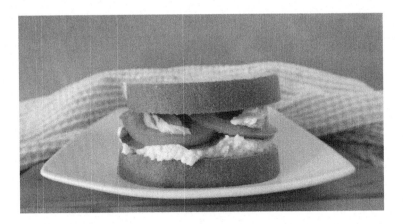

You can use this hummus as a dip, a topping for Buddha bowls and salads, or on a sandwich. One batch makes 2 cups, or 12 heaping tablespoons.

Avocado Bagel

10 Minutes | OF

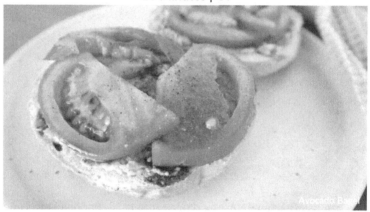

INGREDIENTS:

- 1/2 avocado
- 1 bagel
- 1/2 medium tomato
- 1/2 t sesame seeds
- 1/2 t flax seeds (ground)
- 1/2 t balsamic vinegar
- pepper to taste

INSTRUCTIONS:

Toast the bagel halves if desired. Mash 1/2 avocado with a fork and mix in the ground flax seed. Spread the avocado puree on the two bagel halves, sprinkle with sesame seeds, and top with the tomatoes. Then sprinkle with pepper and drizzle with balsamic vinegar. You can also use your favorite bread and other toppings to make this meal. It is a great no-cook lunch option if you are at work or on the go. This meal is also high in all minerals and vitamin E.

One Bagel: 420 Cal | 64 g Carbs | 7.7 g Fiber | 13.6 g Protein | 13.5 g Fat

Greek Pita With Tzatziki Sauce

10 Minutes

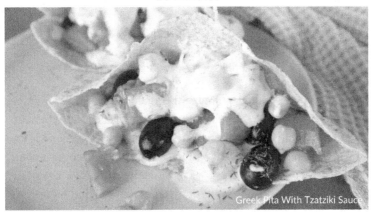

INGREDIENTS:

- Tzatziki Sauce:
  - 1 cup plain plant based yogurt (sugar free)
  - 1/2 cucumber, cubed or shredded
  - juice of 1/2 lemon
  - 1 t garlic powder
  - 1 t dill weed (dried)
  - pepper to taste
- Pita Wrap:
  - 1 pita
  - 1/2 of the tzatziki sauce
  - 10 black olives
  - 1/2 cup (canned, drained, rinsed) chickpeas
  - 1/2 medium tomato (cubed)

INSTRUCTIONS:

Mix all ingredients for the sauce in a bowl. Cut the cucumber into small cubes or shreds. Then cut one pita in half and toast. Open each pita half and add all ingredients. Use 1/2 of the sauce to fill both pita halves. Divide the toppings between both halves. You can adjust toppings to your needs and likes.

One Pita: 510 Cal | 73 g Carbs | 15 g Fiber | 19 g Protein | 19 g Fat

LUNCH AND DINNER RECIPES

NO-COOK LUNCH IDEAS

I typically suggest cooking double the amounts provided for dinner and enjoy the leftovers for lunch the next day. This has two benefits. The first is that you are saving time cooking and the second is that you simply have more recipe options for better meals over multiple days. No-cook meals are typically sandwich based or salads. Sometimes sandwiches are harder to make gluten and oil free and sandwich bread is a processed food.

However, not everyone has the chance to heat up their lunch at work or on the go so there are healthy plant based options. Find no-heat on the go recipe options below:

- Avocado bagel (see sandwich recipes)
- Hummus sandwich (see sandwich recipes)
- Greek pita (see sandwich recipes)
- Burrito (use cold rice, beans, tomatoes, and guacamole in a whole wheat wrap)
- Mexican salad (use the salsa recipe from the Mexican stuffed sweet potato recipe and enjoy as a salad)
- Lentil salad (see salad recipes)
- Caprese salad (see salad recipes)
- Spring roll with peanut dip (use a rice paper wrap and fill with cucumber, spinach, carrots, edamame, or other vegetables. Use the peanut sauce from the peanut sauce stir fry recipe as the dip.

You can still enjoy a warm meal on the go if you take it in a thermos.

Use the one pot meals below and heat one serving in the morning then fill it into a quality thermos to keep warm until lunch time. Each serving is typically 2.5 to 3 cups so make sure your thermos is big enough to hold this amount. Below are all the recipes you can find within this book that are thermos friendly:

- Cauliflower potato stew
- Lemon crema farfalle
- Thai noodle soup
- Mushroom stroganoff
- Creamy tofu tomato linguine
- Easy lentil soup
- Butternut squash ginger soup
- One pot zucchini pasta
- Sweet potato chili
- Creamy coconut potato stew
- Taco elbow pasta
- Creamy pinto bean potato soup

Mexican Stuffed Sweet Potatoes

Serves 4 | 45 Minutes | GF | OF

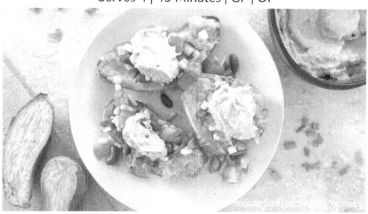

INGREDIENTS:

- 6 medium sweet potatoes
  - **Salsa:**
  - 1 can of corn (or switch for additional beans)
  - 1 can of beans (black or kidney), rinsed, drained
  - 1 bundle spring onion, chopped
  - 1 bundle cilantro (leaves)
  - 3 tomatoes, diced
  - 1 t salt
  - 1 t cumin
  - pepper to taste
  - 2 t red wine vinegar
  - optional: turmeric and pepper
  - **Guacamole:**
  - 2 avocados
  - 1 t onion powder
  - 1 t garlic powder
  - few slices of jalapenos
  - juice of 1 lime

INSTRUCTIONS:

Preheat the oven to 425 F. Wash and slice each sweet potato in half. Place the potatoes on a baking sheet and bake for 25 to 30 minutes. You can poke the sweet potatoes with a fork to see if they are soft. In the meantime prepare the salsa and the guacamole. Add all ingredients for the salsa in a bowl and mix. Then add all ingredients for the guacamole in a blender and mix. You can also use a hand blender. Top each potato with salsa and guacamole. One serving is 3 potato halves. You can remove the corn and add another can of beans for added protein.

Per Serving: 430 Cal | 73 g Carbs | 17 g Fiber | 12 g Protein | 12 g Fat

Creamy Butternut Squash Spaghetti

Serves 4 | 30 Minutes | OF

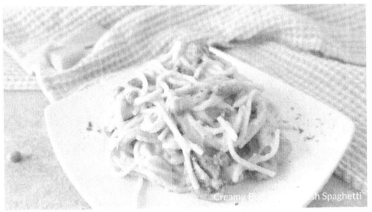

INGREDIENTS:

- 0.5 butternut squash (remove seeds and cut into chunks)
- 4 oz of tofu (any)
- 2-3 cloves garlic
- 2 boxes (or 16 oz) mushrooms, sliced
- 1 cup frozen peas
- 8 oz spaghetti
- 1/2 t onion powder
- 1 t salt

Optional: Add 1/2 cup soaked cashews, 1 t mustard, and more onion powder to the sauce (in the blender) for extra flavor!

INSTRUCTIONS:

Cook the pasta according to package. Steam the butternut squash chunks in 1/2 cup of water until soft, then drain. Steam the sliced mushrooms and the peas with 1/4 cup of water in a third pot until they are done (about 10 minutes) then drain the water. Blend the squash, tofu, garlic, and onion powder in a blender until creamy (you might not need to add water). Add this sauce to the drained pasta and mix in with mushrooms and peas. Add salt and pepper as desired. You can cut the other half of the butternut squash into chunks and freeze for another meal.

Per Serving: 370 Cal | 70 g Carbs | 11 g Fiber | 18.6 g Protein | 3.5 g Fat

Cauliflower Potato Stew

Serves 4 | 25 Minutes | GF | OF | One Pot

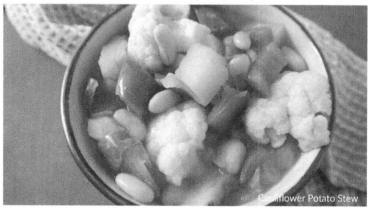

INGREDIENTS:

- 3 medium potatoes, cubed
- 3 green bell pepper, cubed
- 1 head cauliflower, cut apart
- 1 onion, diced
- 2 cans great northern beans (3 cups cooked), rinsed
- 3 cups water
- 2 T paprika powder
- 1 t salt
- 1 t vegetable stock powder
- 2 dashes chili powder

INSTRUCTIONS:

Wash, cut, and prepare all the vegetables. Then add them to one pot or your instant pot. Add the rest of all ingredients. If you cook on the stove (one pot) set heat to medium and cook for 10-15 minutes until potatoes are soft. If you use the instant pot set it to stew, high, 5 minutes and seal the valve. Each serving is about 2-3 cups.

Per Serving: 380 Cal | 77 g Carbs | 18.8 g Fiber | 20 g Protein | 1.3 g Fat

Italian Asparagus Gnocchi

Serves 4 | 20 Minutes | OF

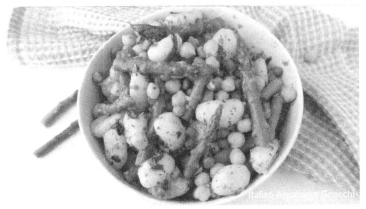

INGREDIENTS:

- 1 can chickpeas (1.5 cups), drained and rinsed
- 1 bundle (4 cups) asparagus, ends removed, cut in 3 parts
- 16 oz. gnocchi (vegan, potato or whole wheat)
- 2 cups frozen peas
- 2 cups fresh baby spinach, chopped
- 3 cloves garlic, pressed
- 2 t Italian herbs
- 0.5-1 t salt
- 1-2 T olive oil (optional)

INSTRUCTIONS:

Cook the gnocchi according to the package (about 3 minutes), then drain. Steam the cut vegetables and chickpeas in 1/2 cup of water for about 10-15 minutes, then drain. Scoop the veggies to the side and create a little circle in the middle of the pan. Add garlic and olive oil and roast for 1-2 minutes on medium heat. If you don't use oil, simply mix in the garlic after draining the veggies and heat for a few minutes. Mix in the gnocchi and all spice. Stir to combine.
The nutritional values includes the use of olive oil.
Read the label when buying gnocchi to make sure it's vegan.

Per Serving: 350 Cal | 50 g Carbs | 11 g Fiber | 14 g Protein | 12.5 g Fat

Fajita Rice Bowl

Serves 4 | 30 Minutes | GF | OF

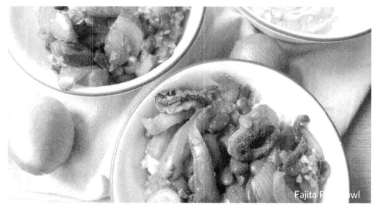

INGREDIENTS:

- 1.5 cups brown basmati rice, dry
- 2 zucchini cut in half and sliced
- 1 box (8 oz) mushrooms, sliced
- 3 green bell peppers, sliced in strips
- 2 cans kidney beans, drained and rinsed
- 1/2 onion, sliced
- juice of 1 lime
- 1 t chili powder
- 1/2 t paprika powder
- 1 t cumin
- 1 t salt
- optional: guacamole to top

INSTRUCTIONS:

Prepare rice according to package. Pour 1/4 cup water to a large pan and add all the veggies and beans. Put the lid on top and let steam on medium heat until soft. Drain remaining water, add the seasoning and lime juice and stir. Use 1 cup rice and top with 1/4 of the fajita mix. You can top your bowl with guacamole if you like.

Per Serving: 460 Cal | 92 g Carbs | 14 g Fiber | 21 g Protein | 4.5 g Fat

Easy Black Bean Mushroom Burger

Serves 4 | 30 Minutes

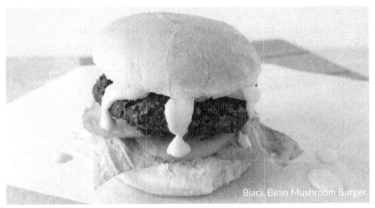

INGREDIENTS:

- 1 box (8 oz) mushrooms
- 1 cup oats (gluten free)
- 2 cans black beans, rinsed
- 1/2 t garlic powder
- 1/4 medium onion
- 1 t paprika powder
- 3 t soy sauce (sodium reduced)
- 1 t flax seed (ground)
- whole wheat buns
- burger toppings

INSTRUCTIONS:

Preheat oven to 400 F. Add one cup of oats into a blender or food processor and grind into powder. Move powder into a larger mixing bowl. Now add mushrooms, onion, and beans in the food processor and chop until small/almost creamy. Combine all ingredients in the mixing bowl and divide mixture into 8 batches. You can press the mass down into the bowl then slice it into 8 pieces like a cake.

Roll each batch into a ball then press down on a baking sheet into a burger patty shape. It should be the size of your burger buns or a bit larger. Leave the patties in the oven for 30-35 minutes but make sure to flip them after about 15 or 20 minutes. The burgers will be crisp on the edges but soft inside. You can adjust the baking time to your desire. Serve on a whole wheat bun and add your favorite toppings. The nutrition mentioned is for 1 serving (2 burgers) with patty and bun, but without the toppings.

Per Serving: 430 Cal | 78 g Carbs | 17.6 g Fiber | 21.2 g Protein | 4.8 g Fat

BURGER SAUCE RECIPE:

The vegan burger sauce you see dripping off the burger is very easy to make. Simply soak 1/2 cup of cashews in warm water for about 15 minutes, then drain. Add 3/4 cup of water with the cashews in a blender and also add: 1/4 tsp. salt, 4 tsp. ketchup, 1/4 tsp liquid smoke, 1 tsp sriracha, 1 tsp vinegar (apple cider), and 1 tsp mustard. You can always add more depending on your taste. Some like it to taste more like mustard, others like to add more liquid smoke or sriracha to spice it up.

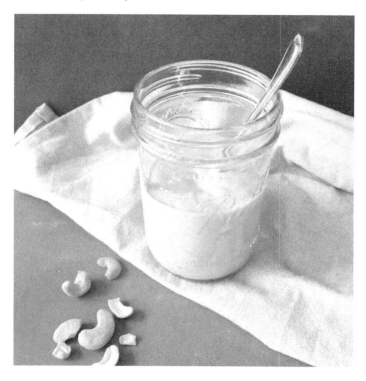

Lemon Crema Farfalle

Serves 4 | 30 Minutes | OF

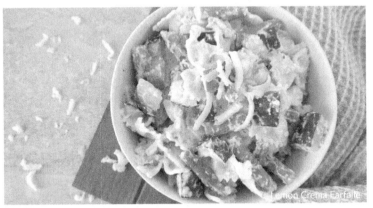

INGREDIENTS:

- 12 oz. dry farfalle pasta (about 4 cups)
- 1 bunch asparagus, cut up (ends removed)
- 3 zucchini, cubed
- 1/2 small onion, diced
- 2 cloves garlic
- 1 lemon
- 8 oz tofu (firm)
- 1/2 cup cashews (soaked in warm water for 10 minutes)
- 2 t rosemary (dried)
- 1 t salt
- pepper to taste

INSTRUCTIONS:

Cover the cashews in warm water and soak for at least 10-15 minutes, then drain. Cook the pasta according to the package, then drain. Steam the asparagus, zucchini and onion in a large pan with about 1/2 cup of water until soft (10 minutes), then drain. To make the sauce, grind off some of the (washed) lemon peel, then squeeze out the juice. Add both (peel and juice) into a blender together with the drained tofu, drained cashews, garlic, salt, and pepper, and blend until creamy. Mix all ingredients together in the large pan and heat up.

Per Serving: 490 Cal | 78 g Carbs | 9 g Fiber | 24 g Protein | 12 g Fat

Thai Noodle Soup

Serves 4 | 20 Minutes | GF | OF | One Pot

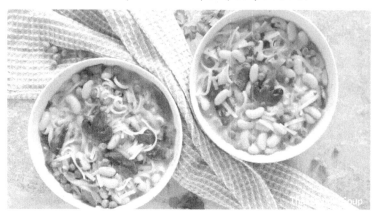

INGREDIENTS:

- 1 can coconut milk, full fat
- 1 bundle cilantro, chopped
- 1/2 onion, chopped
- 2 cloves garlic, pressed
- 2 t vegetable stock powder (optional)
- 3 t soy sauce, low sodium
- 2 can great northern beans
- 1 cups frozen peas
- 16 oz (2 boxes) sliced mushrooms
- 1 lime, juice
- 7 oz rice noodles
- 3 t fresh ginger root, ground
- dashes of turmeric and pepper
- salt (optional)
- 5-6 cups of water

INSTRUCTIONS:

Add 1/4th cup of water to a pot and "fry" the chopped onions and garlic. Then add the rest of ingredients and 5 cups of water to the pot except the pasta. Once the soup is boiling add the pasta and cook for 3-5 minute or as instructed on the pasta package. Add more water if desired.

Per Serving: 500 Cal | 90 g Carbs | 12 g Fiber | 23.5 g Protein | 7.6 g Fat

Peanut Sauce Stir Fry

Serves 4 | 30 Minutes | GF | OF

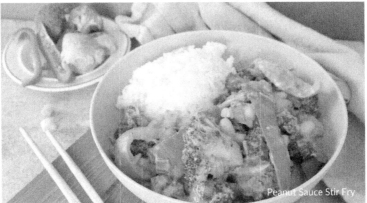

INGREDIENTS:

- 6 heaping tablespoons peanut butter (unsweetened, unsalted)
- 1 T apple cider vinegar
- 1T sriracha
- 3 cloves garlic, pressed
- 4 T soy sauce (sodium reduced)
- 2 T ground fresh ginger
- 1/4 to 1/2 cup warm water
- 1 T maple syrup
- 2 lbs broccoli
- 2 red (or orange/yellow) bell pepper
- 1 bundle green onion
- 2 cans white beans (great northern, drained)
- 1 cup dry rice
- optional: turmeric powder and black pepper

INSTRUCTIONS:

Cook the rice according to the package instruction. Cut and wash the vegetables. Add beans, broccoli, spring onion, and bell pepper to a large pan with 1/2 cup of water and set on medium heat to steam (with a lid). Once the veggies are soft (15 minutes) you can drain the water and add the peanut sauce. For the peanut sauce add peanut butter, apple cider vinegar, sriracha, ginger, soy sauce, garlic, and warm water to a bowl and stir. Add more water if desired. Coat the veggies with the peanut sauce and serve over rice.

Per Serving: 660 Cal | 108 g Carbs | 18 g Fiber | 31.6 g Protein | 14 g Fat

Mushroom Stroganoff

Serves 4 | 20 Minutes | OF

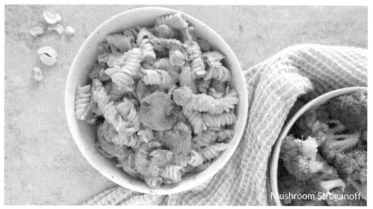

INGREDIENTS:

- 3 boxes of mushrooms, sliced (each 8 oz.)
- 1/2 onion
- 2 cloves garlic
- 1/2 cup cashews, soaked in warm water for 10-15 minutes.
- 1 T soy sauce
- 1/2 t - 3/4 t salt
- 1 t vegetable stock powder (optional)
- 8 oz whole wheat rotini (or other pasta)
- 2 lbs broccoli (side)
- pepper to taste

INSTRUCTIONS:

Cook pasta according to package and soak the cashews in warm water for 15 minutes. Wash and cut broccoli then steam until soft. Wash and slice mushrooms. Fill a pan with 1/4 cup water, add mushrooms and let simmer on medium heat with a lid for about 10 minutes or until the mushrooms are cooked. Then drain mushrooms but save 1/2 a cup of the mushroom water. Add onion, cashews, garlic, salt, pepper, stock powder, 1 cup of mushrooms, and 1/2 a cup of mushroom water to the blender and mix. Combine the sauce, mushrooms, and pasta, and serve with 1/4th of the broccoli on the side. You can also mix in the broccoli if you like.

Per Serving: 540 Cal | 94 g Carbs | 20 g Fiber | 33 g Protein | 11 g Fat

Curried Chickpeas with Water-Fried Potatoes

Serves 4 | 25 Minutes | GF | OF

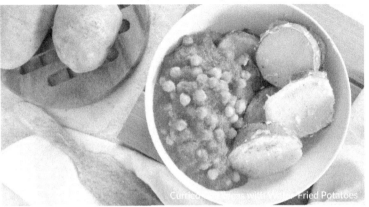

INGREDIENTS:

- 8 potatoes (small, or 4 large)
- 3 bell pepper (red, orange, or yellow).
- 2 cans chickpeas, rinsed
- 1 cup water
- 1/2 onion
- 1-2 clove garlic
- 1 can tomato paste (6 oz.)
- 1/2 t chili powder
- 1/2 t salt
- 1/2 t turmeric + 1 dash black pepper (optional)
- 2 t curry powder

INSTRUCTIONS:

Wash and slice all potatoes (the thinner, the less time they need to cook). You can leave the skin on the potatoes. To water-fry add 1/4 cup to 1/2 cup water to a pan and turn on medium heat. Add the sliced potatoes and a lid. Flip over the potato slices every so often. They should take about 15 to 20 minutes to get soft. In the meantime wash the bell pepper, cut out the core, and cut into larger chunks. Then add them with 1 cup water, garlic, and onion to a blender. Pour this watery mix to a pot and set to medium heat. Add the rinsed chickpeas, tomato paste, and all spices, and stir. Let it heat up thoroughly. After water frying the potatoes you can season them with salt, pepper, and paprika powder, or simply top with the curry.

Per Serving: 550 Cal | 113 g Carbs | 23 g Fiber | 20 g Protein | 4.3 g Fat

Creamy Tofu Tomato Linguine

Serves 4 | 30 Minutes | OF

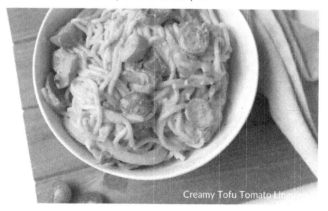

Creamy Tofu Tomato Linguine

INGREDIENTS:

- 1/2 cup cashews, soaked for 10 minutes
- 8 oz. firm tofu
- 2 cloves garlic
- 16 oz tomato sauce
- 1/4 medium onion, chopped
- 1 t basil, dried
- 1 t oregano, dried
- 8 oz dry whole wheat spaghetti
- 2 boxes (16 oz) sliced mushrooms
- 1 pint cherry tomatoes, halved
- salt and pepper optional

INSTRUCTIONS:

Soak the cashews for 10-15 minutes in warm water. Cook the pasta according to package. Before you add the spaghetti to the pot break the strings in half so you can mix it better later. Add tomato sauce, garlic, soaked cashews, tofu, and 1/2 cup water into a blender and mix until creamy. Sauté the onions and mushrooms in 1/4 cup water for 5 minutes in a large pan or pot, then drain the water. In the meantime, cut the cherry tomatoes in half then add them with the rest of the ingredients into the same large pot. Mix well and heat everything thoroughly.

Per Serving: 430 Cal | 66 g Carbs | 10.6 g Fiber | 24.4 g Protein | 12 g Fat

Easy Lentil Soup

Serves 4 | 25 Minutes | GF | OF | One Pot

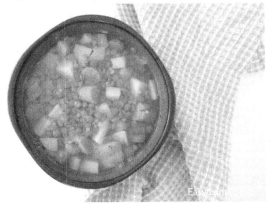

INGREDIENTS:

- 1 cup dry lentils
- 1 clove garlic
- 2 cups diced carrots
- 4 medium potatoes, cubed
- 1 T ground fresh ginger
- 1/2 cup diced onion (or 1 t onion powder)
- 4 stalks celery diced (optional)
- 1 cup riced cauliflower
- 6 cups water
- salt and pepper to taste

INSTRUCTIONS:

Dice everything up as instructed. Add all ingredients with the water to a large pot and cook on medium heat until the potatoes and lentils are soft (about 20 minutes). Add more spices as desired. You can also make this in the instant pot and set to stew - high - 6 minutes. Each serving size equals about 2.5 cups. Double up the serving size and you get 30 g of plant based protein (with 700 calories)!

Per Serving: 350 Cal | 73 g Carbs | 15 g Fiber | 15 g Protein | 1.4 g Fat

Butternut Ginger Soup (or Sweet Potato)

Serves 4 | 30 Minutes | GF | OF | One Pot

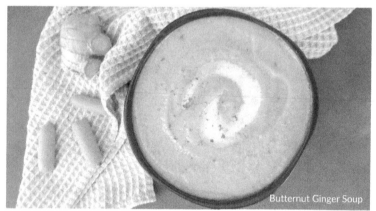

Butternut Ginger Soup

INGREDIENTS:

- 1 butternut squash, cubed (or 4-5 medium sweet potatoes)
- 20 baby carrots
- 2 medium potatoes, cubed
- 1/2 onion, cubed
- 1 t parsley (dried)
- 1 t sage (dried)
- 2 cans great northern beans (3 cups), drained and rinsed
- 1 cup soy milk
- slice of ginger (1 inch, or two if you like it)
- 5 cups water
- hand blender

INSTRUCTIONS:

Bring the water to a boil in a large pot and chop all veggies into larger chunks. Make sure to take the seeds out of the butternut squash and cut off the hard bottom. There is no need to peel the squash. Add all ingredients to the boiling water and cook until they are all soft (about 15-20 minutes). If you use an instant pot you can set it to: stew - high - 5 minutes with a closed valve. Then use a hand blender to puree all ingredients. Add more spices as desired.

Per Serving: 390 Cal | 80 g Carbs | 19 g Fiber | 19 g Protein | 1.5 g Fat

Vegan Sloppy Joe's

Serves 4 | 30 Minutes | One Pot

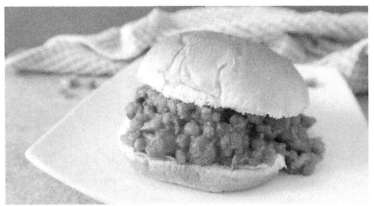

INGREDIENTS:

- 2 cans red lentils (3 cups cooked, 1 cup dry)
- 1/2 onion, chopped
- 1 green bell pepper, chopped
- 2 cloves garlic, pressed
- 2 T tomato paste
- 1 t mustard
- 3 t vegan Worcestershire sauce
- 28 oz (1 large can) diced or crushed tomatoes
- 1-2 t apple cider vinegar (or any other)
- salt and pepper to taste
- Burger buns (whole wheat)

INSTRUCTIONS:

Simply add all ingredients (except the buns) into one pot or instant pot. Cook until the lentils and carrots are soft (about 15 to 20 minutes). If you use the instant pot set to "stew - high - 6 minutes" with a closed valve. Split the meal into 8 parts and serve each part on one bun. One serving equals 2 buns. The nutritional value is only for the sloppy joes mix (not including the bun). You can get a gluten free bun if you like.

Per Serving: 270 Cal | 53 g Carbs | 16.3 g Fiber | 17.8 g Protein | 1.2 g Fat

Roasted Vegetable Sheet Pan (Autumn Version)

Serves 4 | 35 Minutes | GF | One Pan

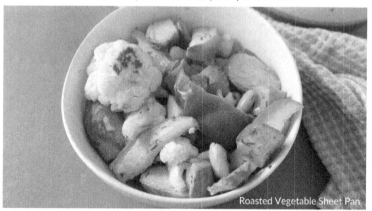

Roasted Vegetable Sheet Pan

INGREDIENTS:

- 1 bag (16 oz) Brussels sprouts, cut in half
- 2 apples, sliced
- 1 onion, diced
- 3 small or medium sweet potato, cubed
- 1 head cauliflower, cubed
- 2 can white beans
- 4 t olive oil
- 1 T apple cider vinegar
- 3 cloves garlic, pressed
- 1/2 T thyme
- 1/2 t salt
- pepper to taste
- large casserole dish or sheet pan

INSTRUCTIONS:

Preheat oven to 400 F. Mix all ingredients in a large bowl, then add the mix to a large casserole dish or sheet pan with parchment paper. Bake in oven for 20-30 minutes until potatoes and Brussels sprouts are soft. Stir the mix a few times. You can also use other vegetables and seasoning for a different taste. For example: During Spring you can use asparagus, broccoli, onion, chickpeas, and more and mix it with Italian herbs instead of the thyme.

Per Serving: 460 Cal | 83 g Carbs | 20 g Fiber | 21.5 g Protein | 8 g Fat

Bean Ball Marinara

Serves 4 | 40 Minutes | OF | GF

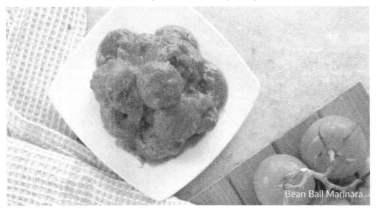

INGREDIENTS:

- 1 can chickpeas
- 1 can black beans
- 1 cup oats
- 1/4 onion
- 2 T flaxseed
- 7 T water (or more)
- 1 cloves garlic
- 1 t basil
- 1 t oregano
- 1/2 t onion powder
- 30 oz tomato sauce
- salt and pepper to taste

INSTRUCTIONS:

Blend the oats in a food processor and set aside. Then add the drained chickpeas and black beans with the onion and flax seed into a food processor and blend into a puree. If it does not blend add one tablespoons of water at the time. I usually add 7 T of water. Blend the mix with the oats and set aside for a few minutes to thicken. Preheat the oven to 450 F. While the oven is preheating you can start rolling the bean balls. If you make medium sized ball you should get 20 bean balls. Bake for 20 minutes on a baking sheet.

Wet your hands or add more oats for better rolling. To make the marinara sauce add the tomato sauce, basil, oregano, onion powder, salt and pepper into a large pan and heat until fully hot. After the bean balls are done you can simply add them to the pot with marinara and stir gently to coat. If the bean balls are too soft, keep them in the oven a bit longer. The nutrition per serving below is for one serving of the bean balls (5 medium balls) and the marinara sauce. If you add one cup of cooked pasta and 2 cups of broccoli you'll get: 516 Cal | 97 g Carbs | 23.6 g Fiber | 26 g Protein | 6.7 g Fat

Per Serving: 245 Cal | 43 g Carbs | 13.4 g Fiber | 12.6 g Protein | 3.6 g Fat

Burrito Bowl with Avocado Lime Crema

Serves 4 | 30 Minutes | OF | GF

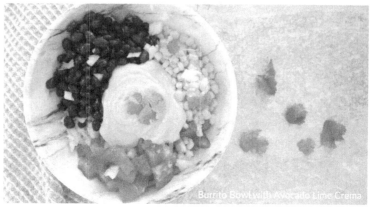

INGREDIENTS:

- 2 avocados
- 1/2 bundle cilantro
- 1 t salt
- 2 t garlic powder
- 2 t onion powder
- 2.5 t cumin powder
- slice jalapenos
- 2 lime, the juice
- 1 cup dry rice
- 1 can corn
- 2 cans black beans (3 cups)
- 1/4 onion, diced
- 4-5 tomatoes, cubed

INSTRUCTIONS:

Cook the rice according to the package. Drain and rinse the corn and beans. Cut the tomatoes, onion, and cilantro. To make the sauce add the avocado (without core and skin) to a blender with the cumin, onion powder, garlic powder, lime juice, jalapenos, salt, and 1.5 cups water and blend until smooth. Now divide all ingredients into 4 servings and prepare your bowl. For a more protein rich bowl you can substitute the rice with quinoa, leave out the corn, add more beans, or use crispy seitan or tofu chunks.

Per Serving: 550 Cal | 95 g Carbs | 22.7 g Fiber | 18.7 g Protein | 13 g Fat

One Pot Zucchini Pasta

Serves 4 | 30 Minutes | OF | One Pot

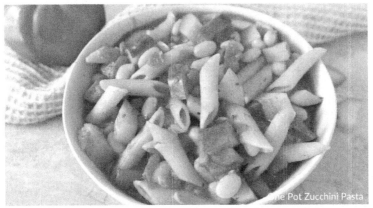

INGREDIENTS:

- 8 oz dry penne pasta
- 1/4 cup water
- 1/4 onion, diced
- 3 cloves garlic, pressed
- 1 T basil (dried)
- 1 T oregano (dried)
- 3 zucchinis, cubed
- 2 cans great northern beans, drained and rinsed
- 2 x 28 oz cans diced tomatoes
- salt and pepper to taste

INSTRUCTIONS:

Add 1/4 cup water to a large pan and add the diced onions and garlic. Water fry for about 3-5 minutes. Then add all other ingredients to the pot and let cook until the pasta is soft (about 20 minutes). Make sure to stir frequently. You can add mores seasoning if you like.

Per Serving: 530 Cal | 105 g Carbs | 18 g Fiber | 28 g Protein | 2.3 g Fat

Sweet Potato Chili

Serves 4 | 30 Minutes | OF | GF | One Pot

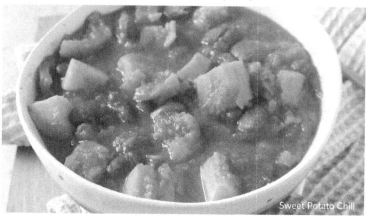

INGREDIENTS:

- 3 green bell pepper, diced
- 1 can (28 oz) crushed or diced tomatoes
- 3 cups / 2 medium sweet potatoes, cubed
- 1/2 onion, diced
- 2 cloves garlic, pressed
- 2 cans kidney beans, rinsed
- 1/2 t salt
- pepper to taste
- 2 t cumin powder
- 1 t paprika powder
- 1/2 t chili powder
- 1 t oregano
- 3/4 cup water
- optional toppings: fresh cilantro, avocado cubes

INSTRUCTIONS:

Add everything into a large pot or instant pot. Let simmer on medium heat until the sweet potatoes are soft (15-20 minutes).

For pressure cooker: Set the instant pot on stew - high - closed valve - 5 minutes. Top with cilantro or avocado for extra flavor.

Per Serving : 426 Cal | 89 g Carbs | 18.8 g Fiber | 18 g Protein | 2.2 g Fat

Creamy Coconut Potato Stew

Serves 4 | 30 Minutes | OF | GF | One Pot

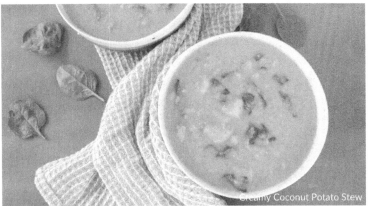

INGREDIENTS:

- 3 bell peppers (red, orange, or yellow)
- 1 can (full fat) coconut milk
- 4 medium potatoes
- 2 cans chickpeas
- 4 oz. (1/2 bag) baby spinach
- 1.5 cups water
- 1 t paprika powder
- 1 t salt
- 4 dashes chili powder
- 4 dashes turmeric powder (optional)
- pepper to taste

INSTRUCTIONS:

Add the coconut milk to a large pot and set to medium-high. Blend 1.5 cups water with 3 bell peppers (core removed) until smooth and add the mixture to the pot. Then wash and cut the potatoes into 1 inch cubes and add to the pot. Once the liquid is boiling, change the heat to medium. Add all the rest of ingredients EXCEPT the spinach and let simmer until potatoes are soft (15-20 minutes). Place a lid on the pot and stir occasionally. You can also make this in your instant pot: stew - high - 5 minutes and closed valve. Once the potatoes are soft use a hand blender and pulse 5-8 times into the mix. This will help make the stew more creamy. Now you can add the spinach and stir until it is wilted.

Per Serving: 540 Cal | 78 g Carbs | 16 g Fiber | 17 g Protein | 17 g Fat

Taco Elbow Pasta

Serves 4 | 20 Minutes | OF | One Pot

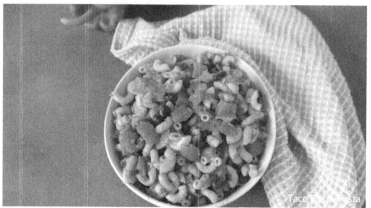

INGREDIENTS:

- 10 oz. dry (whole wheat) elbow pasta (or other small pasta)
- 3 cups veggie stock (or just water)
- 2 cans black beans drained, rinsed
- 2-3 green bell peppers, diced
- 4-5 tomatoes, diced
- 1 taco seasoning mix
- avocado slices (optional)

INSTRUCTIONS:

You can simply add everything into one pot and cook until noodles are soft (about 10 minutes). Add water if desired. You can top your bowl with avocado slices (nutritional value not included). To make this in the instant pot, add all ingredients and set on stew - high - 5 minutes (closed valve).

Per Serving: 450 Cal | 80 g Carbs | 35 g Fiber | 28 g Protein | 1.6 g Fat

Easy Mashed Potatoes

Serves 4 | 30 Minutes | GF | OF

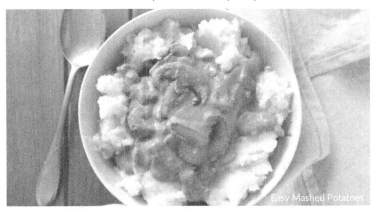

INGREDIENTS:

- 11 small to medium gold potatoes
- 1/4 cup soy milk (unsweetened, original), or cashew milk
- 1/2 t salt
- 1/2 t onion powder
- optional: 1/4 tsp nutmeg

INSTRUCTIONS:

Peel the potatoes and cut into chunks (you can also leave the skin on). Add the potatoes to 1 cup of boiling water and let simmer until the potatoes are soft (about 15 minutes). Drain the water and add the soy milk. Use a potato masher and mash until creamy. Add the seasoning and adjust to taste. You can use the gravy recipe below to top the mashed potatoes, add green veggies on the side, or use this recipe as a side for another dish. Almond milk doesn't make the mashed potato creamy. If you can't tolerate soy you can try cashew, hemp, or oat milk.

Per Serving: 360 Cal | 86 Carbs | 11 g Fiber | 8 g Protein | 0.7 g Fat

Mushroom Gravy

Serves 4 | 20 Minutes | GF | OF

Mushroom Gravy

INGREDIENTS:

- 3 boxes of mushrooms (8 oz each)
- 2/3 cup water
- 1 t vegetable stock powder
- 1/2 cup raw cashews, soaked in water
- 1 t Dijon mustard
- 1 t balsamic vinegar
- 1/2 t onion powder
- 1 t soy sauce, low sodium

INSTRUCTIONS:

Soak the cashews in water for 10 minutes. Slice the mushrooms and add them with the water to a large pan. Cook on medium heat for about 10 minutes. Drain the mushrooms, but save the water in a bowl for later. Now scoop out 1 cup of the cooked mushrooms, and 2/3 cup of the mushroom water. Add the mushrooms and water with the veggie stock powder, cashews, Dijon mustard, balsamic vinegar, onion powder, and soy sauce into a blender and mix until smooth. Add the sauce into the pan with the mushrooms and mix. You can add more of the mushroom water for your desired consistency.

Per Serving: 132 Cal | 11 g Carbs | 2.3 g Fiber | 8.4 g Protein | 7.7 g Fat

Mushroom Bean Balls With Gravy and Rice

Serves 4 | 40 Minutes | GF | OF

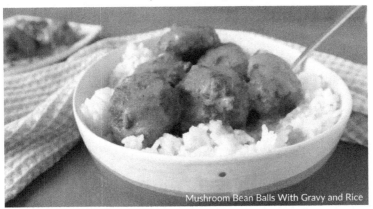

Mushroom Bean Balls With Gravy and Rice

INGREDIENTS:

- Bean Balls:
    - 2 cans black beans, drained (not rinsed)
    - 8 oz. mushrooms
    - 1/4 onion
    - 2 t soy sauce
    - 1.5 cup whole oats
    - 1 t dried thyme
    - 1 T milled flax seed
- Gravy:
    - 1.5 cups water
    - 2 cups soy milk (or cashew milk)
    - 2-3 oz tomato paste (3-5 T)
    - 1 t onion powder
    - 1 t garlic powder
    - 1 T oregano
    - 1 t salt
    - pepper to taste
    - 2 t Worcestershire sauce (vegan)
    - 3 t corn starch
    - optional: dash of nutmeg
    - Rice and broccoli as the side (optional)

INSTRUCTIONS:

Grind the oats into powder and set aside. Blend the beans, onion, and the mushrooms into a puree. If it does not mix, add just a dab of (soy) milk. Now add the bean mix to the oats and stir in the rest of the ingredients until combined. Let sit to thicken for 5 minutes. Preheat the oven to 450 F. Roll small balls (about 30) and put them on a baking sheet. Keep your hands wet for better rolling. Leave the balls in the oven for about 25 minutes. Then transfer them into the gravy and let soak for a few minutes. While the bean balls are baking, steam the broccoli and rice, then make the gravy.

For the gravy, add all ingredients except the cornstarch to a large pan and set to medium-high. Stir frequently. Once the mix is boiling, add the cornstarch: Mix the cornstarch with a bit of water and combine. Make sure there are no clumps in this mix then add it to the gravy to thicken. Adjust as needed. You can also add a splash of wine to this sauce while it is boiling (the alcohol evaporates, but it leaves a great taste). Then turn down the heat and add the bean balls. Split everything into 4 servings (about 7-8 balls per serving) and enjoy! You can leave out the white rice to bring the calories to 450. Adjust this meal to your needs. This recipe makes a large amount of gravy. If you don't eat rice with the meal I suggest cutting the ingredients for the gravy in half.

Per Serving: 650 Cal | 120 g Carbs | 25 g Fiber | 31.7 g Protein | 7 g Fat

Creamy Pinto Bean Potato Soup

Serves 4 | 30 Minutes | GF | OF | One Pot

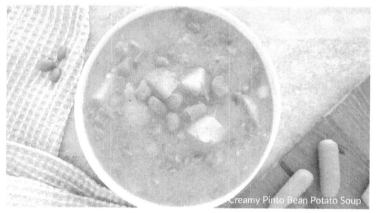

Creamy Pinto Bean Potato Soup

INGREDIENTS:

- 3 cans pinto beans, rinsed
- 4 medium potatoes, cubed
- 4 stalks celery, sliced
- 1 bundle spring onion, sliced
- 2 cups carrots, sliced
- 2 cups spinach
- 1/2 onion, cubed
- 1 t veggie stock powder (optional)
- 2 t Dijon mustard
- 1 t salt pepper to taste
- 5 dashes turmeric
- 4 cups water

INSTRUCTIONS:

Wash everything and cut as described. Place everything except the spinach into a large pot and let simmer until the carrots and potatoes are soft (about 15 minutes). If you use an Instant pot, set to stew - high - 5 minutes with a closed valve. When it is done use a hand blender and press into to the soup 3-5 times. This will make it creamy, but still leaves mostly chunks. Then add the spinach and stir until the spinach is wilted. Add more spices as desired.

Per Serving: 430 Cal | 87 g Carbs | 19.3 g Fiber | 18.6 g Protein | 2.5 g Fat

PART 4: MEAL PLANS

In part 4 you will get several meal plans with meal prep suggestion, shopping list, and meal plan adjustment ideas. Each meal plan can be adjusted to your needs. For example, the weight loss meal plan can also be used for maintenance by increasing serving size or adding another meal to the plan.

You can also customize each meal plan to gluten free by buying gluten free pasta. Smoothies and breakfast recipes are all gluten free. All meal plans are sufficient in protein. I do have an extra high protein meal plan, but all the other meal plans are still high in protein.

The meal plans are also nutritiously sound, meaning you will get enough of all vitamins and minerals as long as you eat all the meals provided. There is no specific "high calcium" or "high iron" meal plan simply because they all contain enough of the minerals. However, if you currently have a deficiency you can add more of the specific nutrient rich foods to the plan. You can view the recommended plant foods in the micronutrient chapter.

Each meal plan has a overview on calories and macro nutrients. Most meal plans serve one person, but can be adjusted to two or more. Just make sure to also adjust the shopping list. The fall/winter meal plan is the only meal plan that serves 2 people. This can also be adjusted to serve one person, but it is a great example how to meal plan for two!

HIGH PROTEIN MEAL PLAN

~2000 Calories | ~123 g Protein | 6 Days

BREAKFAST:

High Protein Smoothie (450 cal, 24 g protein)

LUNCH:

Seitan Pasta With Marinara (600 cal, 51 g protein). The recipe below makes 6 servings. Please make this meal ahead of time and divide into 6 lunch servings for the 6-day meal plan.

Ingredients:

- 16 oz. chorizo seitan
- 16 oz. chickpea pasta
- 2 bunches broccoli
- 3 green bell pepper
- 48 oz vegan marinara sauce

Prepare the chorizo and pasta according to the package. Heat up the marinara then drain the pasta. Mix pasta, marinara, and chorizo together. In the meantime, steam the veggies as the side. Divide everything into 6 servings.

DINNER:

Each recipe serves 4. That means you will eat 2 servings, or half the recipe for one dinner. Make the whole recipe and divide it into two batches. Eat the other half (2 servings) later in the week.

DINNER 1: Thai Noodle Soup, 2 servings (1020 cal, 47 g protein). Make the whole recipe (4 servings) and divide it into 2 parts. Serve the other half of the whole recipe for DINNER 4.

DINNER 2: Taco Elbow Pasta, 2 servings (900 cal, 57 g protein). Make the whole recipe (4 servings) and divide it into 2. Serve the other half of the whole recipe for DINNER 5.

DINNER 3: Vegan Sloppy Joes, 2 servings / 4 buns (860 cal, 46 g protein). Make the whole recipe (4 servings) and divide it into 2. Serve the other half of the whole recipe for DINNER 6.

DINNER 4: 2 Servings (other half) of DINNER 1.

DINNER 5: 2 Servings (other half) of DINNER 2.

DINNER 6: 2 Servings (other half) of DINNER 3.

You can eat a lot of protein on 2000 calories. If you are doing weight exercises you probably have to eat more calories. Easily increase the serving sizes of the meals to increase your calories and protein or add more meals to your plan. Let's say you need 2500 calories, you can simply double up on the lunch and you get around 170 g of plant based protein, without any powder!

Meal Prep:

Pre-cook the lunch and divide it into 6 servings. For the breakfast smoothie, you can place the ingredients for 6 smoothies into 6 jars and each morning add them with the milk to a blender. The one pot meals are also easy meals to prepare ahead of time and freeze.

Shopping List for 1 Person and 6 Days:

6 bananas, 6 cups spinach (baby, fresh), hemp seeds, 8 cups soy milk, 3 cans black beans, dried dates, 16 oz. chorizo seitan, 16 oz. chickpea pasta, 2 bunches broccoli, 6-7 green bell peppers, 48 oz vegan marinara sauce, 1 can coconut milk, 1 bundle cilantro, 1 onion, garlic, soy sauce, 2 cans great northern beans, 1 cup frozen peas, 16 oz. sliced mushrooms, 1 lime, 7 oz rice noodles, fresh ginger, salt, pepper, 3 cups dry elbow pasta, 4-5 tomatoes, 1 taco seasoning mix, 2 cans red lentils (or 1 cup dry), tomato paste, mustard, Worcestershire sauce, 28 oz can crushed or diced tomatoes, apple cider (or other) vinegar, 8 burger buns.

Optional: veggie stock powder, turmeric, avocado slices

WEIGHT LOSS MEAL PLANS

Please note that all the weight loss meal plans can be adjusted to "normal" weight maintenance meal plans. There will be recommendations for each meal plan for increasing calories. Please refer to the calorie section to calculate your caloric needs and make adequate adjustments to your meal plan. You can use any of these examples as inspiration and create your own meal plans as well! Be sure to bookmark, print, or screenshot all recipes and the meal plan for easy access during the week. These weight loss meal plans are designed for one person but you can easily double up on all ingredients to serve 2.

MEAL PLAN FOR BEGINNERS

~ 1750 Calories | ~72 g Protein | 8 Days | GF Option

BREAKFAST:

Easy Balanced Oat Bowl, 1 serving (620 Cal, 18 g protein)

SNACK:

1/8th of the Hummus, 10 baby carrots, 1/2 cup broccoli, and 5 almonds (200 calories, 9.5 g protein). Make the whole batch of hummus and split it into 8 servings. You can prep the hummus beforehand or get store bought hummus (about 800 grams).

LUNCH:

One serving of the dinner from the night before.

DINNER:

Each dinner recipe makes 4 servings. Make each recipe as described in the recipe section then split into 4 equal parts. You can store each serving in meal prep containers during the week. Eat the first serving for dinner and the second serving for lunch the next day. Then repeat this meal later in the week. For example: Make the Fajita rice bowl recipe on the first evening. Eat one serving as dinner 1, the second serving for lunch the next day, the third serving for dinner 5, and the last serving for lunch the next day after dinner 5.

DINNER 1: Fajita Rice Bowl, eat 1 serving (460 cal, 21 g protein)

DINNER 2: Creamy Pinto Bean Potato Soup, eat 1 serving (430 cal, 18.6 g protein)

DINNER 3: Sweet Potato Chili, eat 1 servings (430 cal, 18 g protein)

DINNER 4: Mushroom Stroganoff, eat 1 serving (540 cal, 33 g protein)

DINNER 5: 3rd serving of the fajita rice bowl

DINNER 6: 3rd serving of the creamy pinto bean potato soup

DINNER 7: 3rd serving of the sweet potato chili

DINNER 8: 3rd serving of the mushroom stroganoff

Note: This meal plan starts the evening before Day 1.

	Day 0	Day 1	Day 2	Day 3	Day 4	Day 5	Day 6	Day 7	Day 8
Breakfast		Easy Balanced Oat Bowl, 1 serving	Easy Balanced Oat Bowl, 1 serving	Easy Balanced Oat Bowl, 1 serving	Easy Balanced Oat Bowl, 1 serving	Easy Balanced Oat Bowl, 1 serving	Easy Balanced Oat Bowl, 1 serving	Easy Balanced Oat Bowl, 1 serving	Easy Balanced Oat Bowl, 1 serving
Snack	Grocery shopping	1/8th of the Hummus, 10 baby carrots, 1/2 cup broccoli, and 5 almonds	1/8th of the Hummus, 10 baby carrots, 1/2 cup broccoli, and 5 almonds	1/8th of the Hummus, 10 baby carrots, 1/2 cup broccoli, and 5 almonds	1/8th of the Hummus, 10 baby carrots, 1/2 cup broccoli, and 5 almonds	1/8th of the Hummus, 10 baby carrots, 1/2 cup broccoli, and 5 almonds	1/8th of the Hummus, 10 baby carrots, 1/2 cup broccoli, and 5 almonds	1/8th of the Hummus, 10 baby carrots, 1/2 cup broccoli, and 5 almonds	1/8th of the Hummus, 10 baby carrots, 1/2 cup broccoli, and 5 almonds
Lunch		Fajita Rice Bowl, eat 1 serving	Creamy Pinto Bean Potato Soup, eat 1 serving	Sweet Potato Chili, eat 1 serving	Mushroom Stroganoff, eat 1 serving	Fajita Rice Bowl, eat 1 serving	Creamy Pinto Bean Potato Soup, eat 1 serving	Sweet Potato Chili, eat 1 serving	Mushroom Stroganoff, eat 1 serving
Dinner	Fajita Rice Bowl, eat 1 serving	Creamy Pinto Bean Potato Soup, eat 1 serving	Sweet Potato Chili, eat 1 serving	Mushroom Stroganoff, eat 1 serving	Fajita Rice Bowl, eat 1 serving	Creamy Pinto Bean Potato Soup, eat 1 serving	Sweet Potato Chili, eat 1 serving	Mushroom Stroganoff, eat 1 serving	New meal plan

Calories & Nutrition:

On average you'll get 1750 calories, 72 g protein, 308 g carbs, 61 g fiber, and 37 g fat daily.

You can add the tropical chia pudding to bump your total calories to 2150 and the protein to 81 g. Or you can use the black forest cake smoothie to get more like 2000 calories and 74 g of protein. You can also use any other snack or increase the amount of dinner recipes. Of course, you can also reduce the calories more by removing the snack, but I do not recommend this due to the lack of important nutrients (vitamin A, K, E).

Gluten Free:

To make this meal gluten free use gluten free pasta or rice for the mushroom stroganoff meal. The rest of the meal plan is gluten free. You can also pick another gluten free dinner recipe from the book to replace DINNER 4.

Meal Prep:

You can prep the snacks by filling 8 containers with the veggies and hummus. The hummus lasts at least one week in the refrigerator. The breakfast can also be prepped ahead of time and stored for several days in the fridge. The sweet potato chili and pinto soup can be cooked in the instant pot. All recipes can be stored in the freezer, as well.

Shopping List:

8 cups quick oats, 8 cups almond milk, 4 cups berries (can be frozen), 8 bananas, brazil nuts, chopped walnuts, milled flaxseed, 800g store bought hummus or: 2 cans chickpeas, 1 lemon, garlic, peanut butter or tahini, cumin powder, salt, paprika powder.

3 lbs. baby carrots, 3 lb broccoli, bag of almonds, bag of rice, 2 zucchini, 4x (8 oz) boxes mushrooms (sliced), 6 green bell pepper, 4 cans kidney beans, 2 onion, 1 lime, chili powder, salt, pepper, 3 cans pinto beans, 4 medium potatoes, celery, 1 bundle spring onion, bag of fresh baby spinach, Dijon mustard, 28 oz can crushed or diced tomatoes, 3 large or medium sweet potatoes, dried oregano, cashews, soy sauce (sodium reduced), 8 oz rotini (or other pasta).

Optional: veggie stock powder, turmeric, cilantro (topping), avocado (topping).

NO-COOK LUNCH MEAL PLAN

~1750 Cal | ~82 g Protein | 8 Days

BREAKFAST:

Chocolate overnight oats (410 cal, 19 g protein):

- 0.5 cup oats
- 0.75 cup almond milk
- 1 t peanut butter
- 1 T milled flax seed
- 1 banana
- 1 Brazil nut
- 2 T cocoa powder

LUNCH:

4 Greek Pita (510 cal, 19 g protein): Make 2 batches of the Tzatziki sauce and divide into 4 servings. Make 4 portions of the veggie filling for 4 pitas. Eat 1 Pita per day.

4 servings of the Bean Corn Salad (492 cal, 22.4 g protein). Make one batch (4 servings) and divide into 4 meals:

- 2 cans corn, drained
- 3 cans black beans, drained and rinsed
- 2 avocado
- 7 tomatoes
- 1 bundle spring onion

- 1 bundle cilantro
- 1 t salt
- 2 t cumin
- 3 t red wine vinegar
- pepper to taste

Lunch Prep:

For the salad, chop all veggies and combine them with all ingredients and mix. Then split into 4 equal servings and store in containers. Then prep the sauce for the Pita wraps and divide into 4 servings and store in small containers. Prep all the veggies for the Pita filling and divide them into 4 containers. When you're ready to eat lunch, cut Pita wrap in half then use one serving of veggies and sauce to fill both halves of the Pita. Optional: toast the Pita wrap before filling.

The salad is easy to grab for on the go. Make sure to pack a fork. For the Pita simply pack one Pita wrap, one veggies mix, a sauce, and a spoon. You can dump the veggies and sauce into the wrap right before eating. Don't add this too early or the Pita will get soggy.

DINNER:

DINNER 1: Cauliflower Potato Stew (900 cal, 28 g protein): Cook all 4 servings as described in the recipe and consume 2 servings as one meal. Eat the other 2 servings as one meal for Dinner 5.

DINNER 2: Creamy Tofu Tomato Linguine (850 cal, 48 g protein): Cook all 4 servings as described in the recipe and consume 2 servings as one meal. Eat the other 2 servings as one meal for Dinner 6.

DINNER 3: Sloppy Joes (850 cal, 46 g protein): Cook all 4 servings as described in the recipe and consume 2 servings as one meal (4 buns). Eat the other 2 servings as one meal for Dinner 7.

DINNER 4: Taco Elbow Pasta (890 cal, 57 g protein). Cook all 4 servings as described in the recipe and consume 2 servings as one meal. Eat the other 2 servings as one meal for Dinner 8.

DINNER 5: 2 servings/second half of Dinner 1 (cauliflower potato stew)

DINNER 6: 2 servings/second half of Dinner 2 (creamy tofu tomato linguine)

DINNER 7: 2 servings/second half of Dinner 3 (4 buns of the sloppy joes)

DINNER 8: 2 servings/second half of Dinner 4 (taco elbow pasta)

Calories & Nutrition:

On average you'll eat 1750 calories, 82 g protein, 292 g carbs, 41.5 g fat, and 72 g fiber per day.

If you wish to increase your calories you can change the breakfast recipe above to the full chocolate peanut butter overnight oat recipe found in the recipe section of this book. This will bump the meal plan to around 2000 calories per day and 100 g of protein. You can also cut more calories by only eating one serving for dinner. I don't recommend doing this long term (see calorie and weight loss section).

Meal Prep:

You can make the cauliflower stew, sloppy joes, and the one pot taco pasta in the instant pot. All recipes can be cooked ahead of time and stored in the fridge. Prep the lunches as described and have 8 lunch meals (4 Pitas and 4 salads) ready for the week. The breakfast bowls can be prepped the night before, or in bulk ahead of time.

Shopping List:

4 cup oats, 6 cups almond milk, peanut butter (no salt and sugar added), milled flax seed, 8 bananas, Brazil nuts, cocoa powder, 4 pitas, 2 cups plant based plain yogurt (no sugar added),1 cucumber, 1 lemon, garlic powder, dried dill weed, pepper, salt, can black olives, 1 can chickpeas, 2 cans corn, 4 cans black beans, 2 avocados, 14 tomatoes, 1 bundle spring onion, 1 bundle cilantro, cumin powder, red wine vinegar, 3 medium potatoes, 3 green bell pepper, 1 head cauliflower, 2 onions, 2 cans great northern beans, paprika powder, cashews, 8 oz firm tofu (you can freeze the rest), garlic, 16 oz tomato sauce, dried basil, dried oregano, 8 oz spaghetti, 16 oz mushrooms. 1 pint cherry tomatoes, 2 cans cooked red lentils (or 1 cup dry), 3 green bell pepper, tomato paste, mustard, Worcestershire sauce, 28 oz canned crushed or diced tomatoes, 8 burger buns, box elbow pasta, 1 taco seasoning mix (low sodium).

Optional: chili powder, vegetable stock powder, more avocado for topping (elbow pasta).

SEASONAL MEAL PLANS & FAMILY MEAL PLANNING

These summer and winter meal plans can be used for weight loss depending on your calorie needs. Each meal plan can be adjusted to weight loss, maintenance, or weight gain. The summer meal plan serves one person, while the winter meal plan serves two. You can adjust each plan's serving size and shopping list depending on your family size. The two different options below will give you meal planning ideas. At the end of this chapter you will find tips and tricks for family meal planning, as well.

SPRING/SUMMER MEAL PLAN

~ 1790 Calories | ~67 g Protein | 6 Days

BREAKFAST:

Tropical Sunrise Chia Pudding (400 cal, 14.5 g protein). Make the tropical chia pudding without the soy milk and just top the chia pudding with tropical fruits.

LUNCH:

Caprese Salad (490 calories, 18.2 g protein). Make 2 batches of the recipe and divide the salad equally into 6 meal prep containers.

DINNER:

Each dinner recipe provides 4 servings. Make each dinner recipe as described in the recipe section then split into 2 equal parts. You can store the second serving in meal prep containers for another day of the week.

DINNER 1: Mexican Stuffed Sweet Potatoes (860 cal, 24 g protein). Prep the whole meal (4 servings) and divide into 2 equal parts. Eat one half of the recipe (2 servings are 6 potato halves) and save the other half for Dinner 4.

DINNER 2: Italian Asparagus Gnocchi (712 cal, 28.7 g protein). Prep the whole meal (4 servings) and divide into 2 equal parts. Eat one half of the recipe (2 servings) and save the other half for Dinner 5.

DINNER 3: Lemon Crema Farfalle (980 cal, 48 g protein). Prep the whole meal (4 servings) and divide into 2 equal parts. Eat one half of the recipe (2 servings) and save the other half for Dinner 6.

DINNER 4: Second half of Dinner 1: Mexican Stuffed Sweet Potatoes (6 potato halves)

DINNER 5: Second half of Dinner 2: Italian Asparagus Gnocchi.

DINNER 6: Second half of Dinner 3: Lemon Crema Farfalle.

		Day 0	Day 1	Day 2	Day 3	Day 4	Day 5	Day 6
Breakfast			Tropical Sunrise Chia Pudding	Tropical Sunrise Chia Pudding	Tropical Sunrise Chia Pudding	Tropical Sunrise Chia Pudding	Tropical Sunrise Chia Pudding	Tropical Sunrise Chia Pudding
Lunch		Shopping prep caprese salad for the week	Caprese Salad	Caprese Salad	Caprese Salad	Caprese Salad	Caprese Salad	Caprese Salad
Dinner			Mexican Stuffed Sweet Potatoes (eat half the recipe)	Italian Asparagus Gnocchi (eat half the recipe)	Lemon Crema Farfalle (eat half the recipe)	Mexican Stuffed Sweet Potatoes (eat other half of the recipe)	Italian Asparagus Gnocchi (eat other half of the recipe)	Lemon Crema Farfalle (eat other half of the recipe)

Calories & Nutrition:

This meal plan provides, on average, 1750 calories, 67 g protein, 263 g carbs, 57 g fat, and 60 g fiber daily.

You can increase your caloric intake by adding a smoothie. If you add the grapefruit banana smoothie you'll get 2150 calories and 75 g protein per day. Adjust your shopping list accordingly.

Meal Prep:

You can prep your chia pudding in mason jars or recycled glass jars then top with fruits. It is best to prepare the lunch before you start the week. Simply make 2 batches of the caprese salad recipe then divide into 6 servings and store in the fridge. You can cook the dinners each night or make some ahead of time. You can also pre-cut some of the veggies for shorter cooking time during the week.

Shopping List:

1 bag chia seeds, 5 cups almond milk, 6 cups frozen tropical fruits, 16 oz dry penne or fusili pasta, 3 cans chickpeas, 2 cucumbers, 2 pint cherry tomatoes, 4 avocados, salt and pepper, balsamic vinegar,

dried basil and oregano, 6 medium sweet potatoes, 1 can corn, 1 can black beans, 1 bundle spring onion, 1 bundle cilantro, cumin powder, 3 tomatoes, red wine vinegar, onion powder, garlic powder, 1 jalapenos, 1 lime, 2 bundles asparagus, 16 oz potato gnocchi (vegan), 2 cups frozen peas, fresh baby spinach, garlic, Italian herbs, 12 oz dry farfalle pasta, 3 zucchini, onion, 1 lemon, 8 oz tofu (freeze the rest), cashews.

Optional: olive oil for the gnocchi

FALL/WINTER MEAL PLAN

~1700 Cal | ~70 g Protein | 6 Days | 2 Person

BREAKFAST:

Carrot Cake Oats (530 cal, 20 g protein)

SNACK:

Immunity Boosting Smoothie (250 cal, 5.6 g protein) + 2 T sunflower seeds (added antioxidants / vitamin E)

LUNCH:

Leftover dinner (1 serving per person). You can make the dinner recipes as described to get 4 servings. 2 people would each eat one serving for dinner and the other serving for lunch the next day.

DINNER:

DINNER 1: Creamy Butternut Squash Spaghetti. 1 serving per person (361 cal, 18.6 g protein)

DINNER 2: Sweet Potato Chili. 1 serving per person (426 cal, 18 g protein)

DINNER 3: Butternut Squash Ginger Soup. 1 serving per person (390 cal, 19 g protein)

DINNER 4: Creamy Pinto Bean Potato Soup. 1 serving per person (430 cal, 18.6 g protein)

DINNER 5: Roasted Vegetable Sheet Pan. 1 serving per person (460 cal, 21.5 g protein)

DINNER 6: Cauliflower Potato Stew. 1 serving per person (450 cal, 28 g protein)

	Day 0	Day 1	Day 2	Day 3	Day 4	Day 5	Day 6
Breakfast		Carrot Cake Oats	Carrot Cake Oats	Carrot Cake Oats	Carrot Cake Oats	Carrot Cake Oats	Carrot Cake Oats
Snack		Immunity Boosting Smoothie + sunflower seeds	Immunity Boosting Smoothie + sunflower seeds	Immunity Boosting Smoothie + sunflower seeds	Immunity Boosting Smoothie + sunflower seeds	Immunity Boosting Smoothie + sunflower seeds	Immunity Boosting Smoothie + sunflower seeds
Lunch		Shopping and prep	Creamy Butternut Squash Spaghetti. 1 serving per person	Sweet Potato Chili. 1 serving per person	Butternut Squash Ginger Soup. 1 serving per person	Creamy Pinto Bean Potato Soup. 1 serving per person	Roasted Vegetable Sheet Pan. 1 serving per person	Cauliflower Potato Stew. 1 serving per person
Dinner		Creamy Butternut Squash Spaghetti. 1 serving per person	Sweet Potato Chili. 1 serving per person	Butternut Squash Ginger Soup. 1 serving per person	Creamy Pinto Bean Potato Soup. 1 serving per person	Roasted Vegetable Sheet Pan. 1 serving per person	Cauliflower Potato Stew. 1 serving per person	New meal plan...

Calories & Nutrition:

One person consumes 1690 calories, 65 g protein, 293 g carbs, 33 g fat, and 61 g fiber daily. You can increase the serving sizes to your needs. If you do so, make sure to also change the shopping list.

Meal Prep:

You can prep all overnight oats beforehand in food containers and store in the fridge. The smoothie ingredients can also be prepped and stored in glass jars. You can then mix the smoothie in the morning and use the jar as a to go cup. All soups can be made in the instant pot. All meals can be frozen or cooked ahead of time.

Shopping List for 6 Days and 2 People:

9 cup whole quick oats, 5 lbs. baby carrots, chia seeds, chopped

walnuts, cinnamon, 13 cups soy milk, (optional: maple syrup, turmeric powder, avocado and cilantro topping, vegetable stock powder, olive oil for roasting veggies), vanilla extract, nutmeg, raisins, Brazil nuts, 14 apples, 12 oranges, 2 bags of baby spinach, unsalted cashews, black pepper, ginger, 1.5 butternut squash, 4 oz of tofu, garlic, 2 boxes (16 oz) mushrooms, 1 cup frozen peas, 8 oz spaghetti, 3 onions, onion powder, salt, 6 green bell pepper, 1 can (28 oz) crushed or diced tomatoes, 5 sweet potatoes, 2 cans kidney beans, cumin, paprika powder, chili, oregano, cilantro, 9 potatoes, parsley, sage, 6 cans great northern beans, 3 cans pinto beans, 4 stalks celery, 1 bundle spring onion, Dijon mustard, 1 bag (16 oz) Brussels sprouts, 2 head cauliflower, apple cider vinegar, thyme.

KID FRIENDLY FAMILY MEAL PLANNING

Family meal planning can be a bit more challenging. You have to make meals that everyone in your family loves while, at the same time, tracking your nutrition to reach your health and weight goals. Below are recipes and meal ideas that are toddler approved and kid friendly.

You can create your own meal plan that fits your family's needs. Of course, you can try new and different recipes. I simply summarized some meal ideas based on my personal experience. In Phase 1 – Challenge 1 you can read more about how to eat plant based with your partner and kids.

BREAKFAST IDEAS:

- Simple oats with flax seed and fruits
- Oat waffles with jelly or maple syrup and fruit on the side
- Bran flakes/raisin bran cereal with fruits (carefully review label of bran flakes)

SNACK:

- Breakfast smoothie
- Apples with peanut butter
- Cucumber and baby carrots with hummus
- Chickpeas
- Chips and guacamole (from the stuffed sweet potato recipe)
- Dried fruits
- Nuts
- Chocolate chips
- Fruits with vegan chocolate sauce or melted vegan chocolate
- Pretzels
- Whole grain crackers dipped in apple sauce (no added sugar)
- Puffed rice cakes with peanut butter (or other nut butter)
- Air fried vegetable chips
- Banana sushi
- Vegan yogurt (watch sugar content)

Notes: Let your child try different nut types. Some might be more favorable. You can find vegan chocolate and chocolate sauce in most grocery stores. They are not labeled vegan, so be sure to read the label. For the banana sushi spread peanut butter over a tortilla, roll the banana into it, then cut into "sushi" chunks.

COLD LUNCH IDEAS:

- Sandwich with homemade hummus and favorite vegetables
- English muffin/with peanut butter and jelly
- Burritos with beans, tomatoes, guacamole (or other toppings)
- Hummus quesadilla (tortillas with hummus spread)
- Peanut butter jelly quesadilla

DINNER RECIPES:

I know children can be very picky. It is important to determine which vegetable he/she likes. I take out ingredients separately when I know my child doesn't like the sauce. I will serve rice, beans, and veggies only. For stews, I know my child does not like the soup consistency so I take out the food he likes and put it on a plate. The pasta dishes with creamy sauces are a favorite. I use cashews mixed with veggies (cauliflower, butternut squash, mushrooms) to make a cream sauce. Sometimes I blend in some tofu or beans for added protein. You can start with these recipes, but your child might surprise you and like more "exotic" foods, as well. Therefore, it is always a good idea to try new foods and introduce different plant foods here and there. Here are some recipes to start with:

- Mashed potatoes with beans and veggies
- Thai noodle soup (without much of the liquid, make it more like a pasta meal)
- Fajita rice bowl (pick out the veggies and beans your kid likes)
- Taco elbow pasta
- Cauliflower potato stew (take out the veggies and beans that the kid likes)
- Peanut sauce stir fry (might want to leave out the hot spices)
- Lemon crema farfalle (this could be hit or miss)
- Mushroom stroganoff

- Sweet potato chili
- Creamy tofu tomato linguine
- Bean balls with marinara and spaghetti
- Burrito bowl with child's favorite toppings

If you have a family of 4, you can easily make the recipes that serve 4. The meal sizes in this book are medium sized. It can get tricky when the rest of the family likes to eat larger portion sizes. In this case you can cook double the amount of food and simply measure out your portion size for better calorie counting. A typical serving size for my recipes is 2.5 to 3 cups. You can take your serving size out on a plate or in a food container then serve the rest to the family.

Thank you for reading this book. I hope it helped you take a step into plant based eating. Share your thoughts and review! For any questions contact me at www.2sharemyjoy.com/contact.

Acknowledgments

Thank you to all the followers and readers of my website 2sharemyjoy.com. Your emails and questions have inspired me to write this detailed vegan nutrition book. Because of your feedback and motivation this book will help many others to transition into a healthy plant based diet.

A big thank you to my friends and family who encouraged me to write this book and those that shared my excitement when I completed this work. I'm not going to lie, it has been a lot of work! Thank you for reviewing this book and providing your insight.

To my husband, Terry: Thank you for enduring many recipe fails, always encouraging me, and sharing your experience with the vegan diet.

Another thank you to my dear friend and nutrition scientist Lisa Ferrari: You have enriched this book greatly with your knowledge. I appreciate your honesty, expertise, and time.

Resources

For my newest vegan recipes and nutrition tips, visit 2sharemyjoy.com

Nutrition Facts (Dr. Greger):

nutritionfacts.org

Barnard Medical Center:

www.pcrm.org/barnard-medical-center

Dr. Joel Kahn:

www.drjoelkahn.com

Moving Medicine Forward:

www.doctorklaper.com/moving-medicine-forward

The China Study:

nutritionstudies.org/the-china-study

Dr. Esselstyn:

www.dresselstyn.com/site

Forks Over Knives:

www.forksoverknives.com

The Game Changers (Documentary):

gamechangersmovie.com/getting-started

What The Health (Documentary):

www.whatthehealthfilm.com/take-action

About The Author

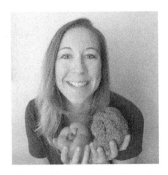

Lisa Goodwin is the creator of the website 2 Share My Joy, where she shares vegan nutrition and weight loss tips, easy plant based recipes, and meal plans. Her website started out with non-vegan budget recipes in 2016. When she switched to a plant based diet in 2018, her blog took a big turn. Her recipes have been featured on many popular sites including Women's Health Magazine.

She dedicates her time researching vegan nutrition and experimenting with new vegan recipes to ensure her family receives adequate nutrition. Each family member enjoys all of the featured easy, budget friendly recipes.

Lisa grew up in Germany where she earned her degree at the University of Saarland in Education, Sports, and Theology. She currently lives in the United States with her husband, son, and two dogs. As a nutrition nerd, she earned her certification in Vegan Nutrition. You can find more of her work on the website www.2sharemyjoy.com

Made in the USA
Columbia, SC
26 April 2021